KETO DIET COOKBOOK FOR WOMEN AFTER 50

Over 200 Quick, Simple and Delicious Recipes For Women Undergoing Hormonal Changes And Struggling To Get Back Into Shape. Including A 28-Day Meal Plan.

Lisa Riggins

TABLE OF CONTENTS

INTRODUCTION

Are you over 50 years old and looking for a weight loss solution? You can achieve this by following one of the most popular diets—the Keto diet. The Keto diet will help you burn excess fat and retrieve your youth. Also, you won't feel starved when dieting anymore. The Keto diet allows you to eat meats and fats, and you'll feel satiety with no guilt. You may wonder why the Keto diet is so magical.

Face it – we all struggled with weight problems at some point in our life. In fact, some people still struggle with weight loss and would happily lose a few more pounds, if given the chance.

To offset this change, there is a need to increase the amount of protein in the diet. At the same time, bone density decreases, making it necessary to increase the amount of vitamin D and calcium consumed in order to maintain adequate bone density as the body ages. All this, combined with a reduction in the number of calories needed to fuel the body, makes it necessary to modify diet as a woman enters postmenopausal years. These natural changes to the body make changes to the diet necessary as a woman ages.

Because of the changes occurring in the bodies of women over 50, it is imperative to look at how the needs of these women are different than younger women and men. During menopause, hormones shift in women, and these changes make it necessary to make some adjustments to their lifestyle in general, and diet in particular.

Also, as women age, their ability to discern thirstiness may diminish. Water consumption is still an important factor in the health of a woman. Because it is harder to determine thirst as you surpass your 50th year, it is essential that you consume 8 to 9 8 oz glasses of water each day. Drink more in the winter in hot weather and when exercising. While you are drinking more water, it may serve to curb your appetite. This is good because you will need to lower your caloric intake from what you may be accustomed to. This happens when you are finding new aches and pains and slowing down your exercise regime. Exercise may be less intense as you make modifications to coincide with your age and decreases in mobility. This is because you are not as flexible and may be experiencing inflammation in your joints. While these are all relatively normal signs of aging, the decrease in physical activity may cause additional problems in the form of weight gain.

This may be a good time to eliminate processed foods and sugar from your diet. Dietary fiber is the key to avoiding constipation.

In this book, I've made every effort to communicate what I know and have learned after years of enjoying the benefits of the Ketogenic Diet. If you've read Keto books before and became frustrated about the in-depth and complicated explanations – don't worry anymore! I've made sure that this book is as simple and as straightforward, giving you only what is considered essential in order to make the most out of the Ketogenic Diet.

But that's enough talking – read on and find out exactly what you can enjoy even as you enter your older years!

This is a beginner's guide to successfully maintaining a Keto diet, as a woman over the age of 50-years-old. Over the last few years, you have likely heard a lot about the Keto diet. It is known as being a diet that allows you to indulge, while still promoting weight loss. People of all ages have seen its incredible benefits.

Keto is different and this guide will show you all the reasons why. It is an overall lifestyle change that is possible for almost everyone, no matter what your average day looks like. You will be filled with plenty of optimism and all the positivity necessary in order to meet your goals. Whether you want to maintain your current weight or lose weight in the process, Keto will help you get to where you truly want to be. It will become an anti-aging diet that will ultimately be a regular part of your everyday life.

If you are ready to feel great and look great, then you are ready to begin your own Keto diet. It will be a diet like no other because you will feel great every step of the way. There are no tricks or deceiving steps that you must take in order to succeed with the diet. If you are educated on what you need to be eating, you should have no problem incorporating the Keto diet into your current lifestyle. So, let's jump in and learn about the Keto diet, and how it can help you!

Be patient and overcome those obstacles. At the end of the tunnel, the reward is too outstanding to give up on.

This book will open the door of the Keto diet for you and lead you on the right path to a healthy lifestyle. What are you waiting for? Let's explore it together!

CHAPTER 1:

Is the Ketogenic Diet Healthy?

What Is the Ketogenic Diet?

The Ketogenic Diet follows a simple principle: keep your food consumption low-carb and high-fat. So basically, being on the diet means eating less carbohydrates and adding more fats in your daily meals. Don't be confused. When we say "fat" we're not talking about the literal kind that's attached to your body. Fat has gotten a bad reputation nowadays, but "fat" the nutrient is actually very different from the "fat" that makes your clothes fit tight.

Good fats are the kind you get from avocado, nuts, and fish. For example, there are the omega-3 and omega-6 fatty acids that actually help you lose weight, get better heart health, and have excellent hair and nails.

A keto diet is a pattern of eating which is an intake of high fat, moderate protein and low crabs which is different from the general pattern of eating you cannot have all the health items in your plate because they contain carbs including fruit, vegetables, whole grains, milk, sugar, yogurt. And you can eat proteins like eggs, meat, cheese, and some of your favorite things which might be a cheat meal for other diet plans.

Carbs of all types are limited but you can decide how much quantity you want to take for keeping underneath 50 grams every day.

For what reason does the Keto diet limit carbs?

So here you think about restricting carbs in your diet either it's a fruit or the vegetables.

Fruits and vegetables also contain many of the healthy nutrients not just carbs so what carbs do to your body that restricting carbs will help you in shedding stubborn pounds.

The body also uses ketones as an alternative energy source for the brain. Hence, the name for this eating pattern.

What Happens to Your Body When You Eat Keto?

Even before we talk about how to do keto – it's important to first consider why this particular diet works. What actually happens to your body to make you lose weight?

As you probably know, the body uses food as an energy source. Everything you eat is turned into energy, so that you can get up and do whatever you need to accomplish for the day. The main energy source is sugar so what happens is that you eat something, the body breaks it down into sugar, and the sugar is processed into energy. Typically, the "sugar" is taken directly from the food you eat so if you eat just the right amount of food, then your body is fueled for the whole day. If you eat too much, then the sugar is stored in your body – hence the accumulation of fat.

But what happens if you eat less food? This is where the Ketogenic Diet comes in. You see, the process of creating sugar from food is usually faster if the food happens to be rich in carbohydrates. Bread, rice, grain, pasta – all of these are carbohydrates and they're the easiest food types to turn into energy.

So, the Ketogenic Diet is all about reducing the amount of carbohydrates you eat. Does this mean you won't get the kind of energy you need for the day? Of course not! It only means that now, your body has to find other possible sources of energy. Do you know where they will be getting that energy? Your stored body fat!

So, here's the situation – you are eating less carbohydrates every day. To keep you energetic, the body breaks down the stored fat and turns them into molecules called ketone bodies. The process of turning the fat into ketone bodies is called "Ketosis" and obviously – this is where the name of the Ketogenic Diet comes from. The ketone bodies take the place of glucose in keeping you energetic. As long as you keep your carbohydrates reduced, the body will keep getting its energy from your body fat.

Sounds Simple, Right?

The Ketogenic Diet is often praised for its simplicity and when you look at it properly, the process is really straightforward. The Science behind the effectivity of the diet is also well-documented and has been proven multiple times by different medical fields. For example, an article on Diet Review by Harvard provided a lengthy discussion on how the Ketogenic Diet works and why it is so effective for those who choose to use this diet.

Positive and Negative Effects of Keto

When you hear a person is on diet, what do you think the primary reason is?

Yes, they want to lose weight, and this is the primary benefit of any diet including the keto diet so when someone decided to lose some of the pounds or fit into their dream outfit, they start the diet. Keto diet helps in losing the weight there are many other benefits of keto diet the proven facts but some of the side effects also except burning fat it controls appetite and this is true while you are on a keto diet you see many positive results that all the dieters usually notice.

Ketones that provide more energy to the body than glucose and keto diet helps in improving stamina, physical fitness, and performance. With all the proven benefits, they also have some negative effects.

Physical Benefits:

- Improved physical performance

- Weight Loss

- Lowered risks of metabolic syndrome and cardiovascular disease

- Lowered blood sugar, triglycerides, and bad cholesterol levels

- Better immune system

- Balanced hormone levels

- Slow aging process

- Reduced inflammation

- Increased metabolism

- Psychologically help as

- Help and enhanced brain function

- Improvement in autistic cases

- Reduced episodes of epilepsy

- In Alzheimer's patients, there is an improvement in cognitive function

- Reduce bipolar disorder's symptoms

So, here are all the benefits of keto diet. These are all the positive changes that a keto diet can bring in your life and it can surely change many things physically, keep your heart healthy, lower cholesterol, lower blood pressure, and surprisingly can help you in many psychological disorders. It also improves skin by reducing acne.

All these benefits are mostly proven but here come some risks which can also be even fatal for one's life if we ignore them. Everyone's need for daily diet is different and some of the side effects which appeared in people some side effects are common and some are not, but all of these side effects still need to be addressed.

Negative Effects of Keto Diet

Keto Flu

The very first symptom which appears when someone start a keto diet is keto flu. This is a phase from 1 day to 2 weeks for your body to adjust with ketosis because when you suddenly leave all the carbs and change your whole diet by adding more fat and proteins the restriction of carbs for the body is a new phase and it takes some time to adjust with ketosis sometimes it only takes a week sometimes more but it is a short term phase.

As everything has its drawback, with a lot of the benefits in keto diet some of the side effects are present and these are all with the short span of their symptoms, but there is no such case till now with the extremes, however it can be fatal for the patients with diabetes 1. The reason is the use of Insulin and their medication except that more benefits are there which we can get through following a keto diet and some of the people who started it used as a diet plan for few days ended up adopting it as there lifestyle.

All meals including breakfast, lunch, dinner, with one or two snacks in a day with the keto diet does not feel like a diet because there is no restriction for the fats like cheese or eggs which are already a very important part of your life and are your favorite foods.

How to get into Ketosis

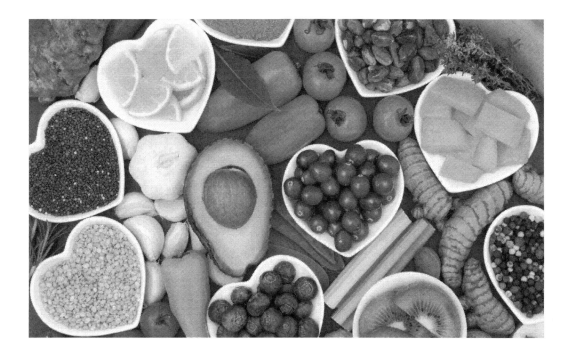

The process of burning fat from your body by reducing your carbohydrate intake is understood as losing weight by ketosis. Within the past 10 years approximately, we've heard mention of the Atkins diet which is predicated on the ketosis process.

A low carbohydrate diet uses ketosis or better said ketosis is how you experience weight loss from the low carbohydrate diet.

When there's an absence of sugar and glucose within the bloodstream your body will produce ketones for energy. This is often what the Atkins diet is all about. When your body is creating ketones, this is often referred to as ketosis. At the arrival of the Atkins diet, people were saying that following a ketogenic diet was harmful to your health when actually it's a wild when your body is creating ketones for energy because there's no sugar or glucose available.

The reason you're dieting is that there's an absence of exercise and activity in your lifestyle. Exercise isn't really instrumental within the ketosis process, i'm inserting this reminder here that no matter what your weight-loss objective is or what goals you would like to realize, you would like to possess an exercise regime. You ought to develop this regime as a part of a healthy lifestyle which can cause an extended and meaningful life.

How to know you are in ketosis

During a ketogenic diet, our body shows various signs and symptoms which confirms that your body is in the metabolic state known as ketosis. Some signs and symptoms are as below:

Rapid Weight loss

when our body enters the ketosis state. Due to the low-carb diet glycogens store are decrease rapidly from your body. These glycogens are mostly of water; one molecule of glucose holds three molecules of water. Due to this, you lose your water weight rapidly. Losing weight during the ketogenic diet is a good sign that ensures that you are into ketosis.

Bad Breath

This is one of the common signs occurs during the process of fat breaking. In this process acetones are released from the mouth due to this you have to face bad breath problems during the diet. Acetone is used by nail polish maker it smells like gasoline, fruity and sweet. This problem basically occurs during the first week of the ketogenic diet. It goes away after some weeks during the keto diet. This problem is not happening with everyone it is one of the common side effects of ketosis. This is one of another good signs indicates that your body is in the state of ketosis.

Dry Mouth and Increased Thirst

During the diet, most people feel thirstier than usual. This may occur because of carb restrictions and the production of ketones. Due to this your body rapidly loses water and the body leads to dehydration. One of the reasons is that when you are in ketosis your body insulin level decreases. Due to this, your kidney releases sodium and water from your body. This is one of the signs indicates that your body is in the state of ketosis.

Increased Focus and Energy

Long term ketogenic dieters notice that increase in focus and energy. When you are in the ketosis your body burns fats for energy instead of glucose. Instead of glucose, your brain burns ketones for energy. This is happening due to stable blood sugar levels and more stable energy levels because of increased ketone levels. This is also a good sign indicates you are in the state of ketosis.

Increase Urination

Increase frequent urination due to a decrease in body insulin level and your body release more sodium and water. When you are in ketosis your body losses glycogens from the body these glycogens hold 3 to 4 parts of water in it. Due to this urination is increased during ketosis. This is one of the good signs ensures that your body is in the state of ketosis.

Insomnia

This problem is occurring when you are adopting the keto diet the first time. You are having trouble to fall asleep at night. Ketogenic diet interrupts a person's sleeping habits. This insomnia symptom typically is gone within some weeks of the ketogenic diet.

CHAPTER 2:

What Does the Ketogenic Diet Mean to Women After 50?

Body Changes after 50

The endocrine system is the body's system that produces hormones. Hormones are potent chemicals that convey messages through the body to regulate certain processes. Hormones are needed for growth, fertility, metabolism, the immune system, and a person's mood or behavior.

As we age our hormones change and our body produces more of some, less of others. Hormones are produced in accordance with the person's stage of life. For example, a teenager's hormones are produced to get them through puberty. The following stage of development for the human body where hair starts to develop in strategic places. A woman's body changes and starts to get ready for the subsequent stage, which is to produce offspring.

During pregnancy, the body produces the human chorionic gonadotropin (HCG) hormone. As well as human placental lactogen (HPL) hormone, estrogen, and progesterone. As most people know, women seem all over the place both physically and emotionally when they are expecting. Now you know why with all these extremely potent chemicals being produced.

Women go through perimenopause usually during their mid-forties. At this stage, the body's estrogen production starts to slow down until they go through menopause. During menopause, the body stops releasing eggs which means a woman is no longer able to reproduce.

Most women will go through menopause between the ages of fifty-one to fifty-two. It can last anywhere from one to three years and the symptoms of menopause can include:

The menstrual cycle has stopped for a year or more.

Problems sleeping.

Bad night sweats that can drench a person.

Uncomfortably dry or itchy skin that feels like you have a thousand ants crawling on you. Problems with urination like releasing little drops when sneezing, problems urinating, and incontinence issues.

Urinary tract infections or dryness which leaves a burning sensation.

Decreased libido and disinterest in intimacy.

Some women experience varying degrees of lethargy.

Hot flashes that cause a person to feel like the doors of hell have opened in front of them. These come on suddenly with no warning at any time or place during the day.

Some women will experience all these symptoms, some of them, and others may get them more mildly or not at all. Menopause and its symptoms are a lot like being pregnant without giving birth at the end. The hormones or lack thereof, affect each woman differently. It wholly depends on how your body adjusts to the current phase in its lifecycle.

It is vital to try and balance your hormones. One hormone which increases when practicing intermittent fasting is the growth hormone. As soon as a person stops eating for long enough, the body starts to produce this hormone. It is the hormone sent out to repair tissue and is typically called the fountain of youth hormone due to its reparative qualities. While it doesn't do much to change menopause, it will help slow down the aging process and help you retain muscle. It also helps with weight loss, and intermittent fasting has been shown to almost double this hormone in the body.

During menopause, two hormones that become imbalanced are melatonin and cortisol. These are the hormones that need to be in sync, as melatonin helps a person sleep and enjoy good quality sleep. While cortisol is the hormone that helps a person wake up, feel alert, and keep the mind clear. An imbalance of these two hormones is usually due to a health problem, anxiety, stress, and menopause. Intermittent fasting along with proper nutrition may aid in the production and balance of these two hormones.

Homeostasis is the term used for hormone balance and it is vital for optimum health. To be successful with an intermittent fasting program, you also need a nutritious diet. Once a woman reaches fifty it is imperative to live a healthy lifestyle to ensure you enjoy your golden years in peak form.

Women over fifty should strive to:

- Eat well but healthily and make smarter food choices.

- Fast within their comfort zone and make it a part of their life.

- Take supplements to ensure they are getting enough vitamins and minerals.

- Take care of their skin by implementing the proper treatments in or out of the sun.

- Wear protection in the heat when outside. Wear a hat to cover your face and neck. Wear sun protection, although a good 15 minutes of direct sunlight will increase vitamin D.

- Exercise at least two to three times a week, more if you can.

- Most importantly drink lots of water.

For women over 50, there are guidelines to follow when you start your Keto diet. As long as you are following the method properly and listening to what your body truly needs, you should have no more problems than men do while following the plan. What you will have are more obstacles to overcome, but you can do it. Remember that plenty of women successfully follow a Keto diet and see great results. Use these women as inspiration for how you anticipate your own journey to go. On the days when it seems impossible, remember what you have working against you, but more importantly what you have working for you. Your body is designed to go into ketogenesis more than it is designed to store fat by overeating carbs. Use this as a motivation to keep pushing you ahead. Keto is a valid option for you and the results will prove this, especially if you are over the age of 50.

This isn't going to be fun to read but once you hit your 50s, you're likely to experience a number of changes in your body. The most common include:

<u>Weight Gain</u>

According to Centers for Disease Control and Prevention (CDC), men and women are likely to gain one to two pounds each year as they transition from adulthood to middle age. This doesn't get any better for women as they hit menopause. While gain in belly fat isn't directly linked to menopause, hormonal changes may cause you to pack a few pounds, depending on lifestyle and environmental changes.

<u>Metabolism Slows Down</u>

You've probably heard a lot about your metabolism changing as you grow older. That's probably why you can't chow down junk food like you used to when you were in your teens. So, what is metabolism and how does it affect your body?

In simple terms, metabolism is how quickly your body processes or converts food and liquids into energy. As you grow older, metabolism slows down and the body starts to convert those extra calories into fat. This is probably why you should skip those convenience meals and start to eat healthier.

Why Should You Switch to Keto?

Once you start to hit 50, you likely don't indulge in strenuous activities anymore which is why you'll be needing fewer calories to function. This is when you should start eliminating added sugars from your diet. In addition, most packaged meals or meals provided in the hospital for the elderly are processed and contain empty calories including mashed potatoes, bread, pastas, and puddings. Not only do these foods taste bland but they also lack nutrition to keep your body strong and healthy.

Plus, a low-carb diet that is rich in healthy vegetables and meat will prove to be far better for folks suffering from insulin insensitivity and your overall health. Hence, start reading food labels more often and opt for healthier options. A recent study from the Hebrew University of Jerusalem has indicated how eating a diet rich in healthy fats can help you lose weight in the long run.

Ketogenic Diet and Menopause

For ageing women, menopause will bring severe changes and challenges, but the ketogenic diet can help you switch gears effortlessly to continue enjoying a healthy and happy life. Menopause can upset hormonal levels in women, which consequently affects brainpower and cognitive abilities. Furthermore, due to less production of estrogens and progesterone, your sex drive declines, and you suffer from sleep issues and mood problems. Let's have a look at how a ketogenic diet will help solve these side effects:

Enhanced Cognitive Functions

Usually, hormone estrogen ensures the continuous flow of glucose into your brain. But after menopause, the estrogen levels begin to drop dramatically, so does the amount of glucose reaching the brain. As a result, your functional brainpower will start to deteriorate. However, by following the keto diet for women over 50, the problem of glucose intake is circumvented. This results in enhanced cognitive functions and brain activity.

Hormonal Balance

Usually, women face major symptoms of menopause due to hormonal imbalances. The keto diet for women over 50 works by stabilizing these imbalances such as estrogen. This aids in experiencing fewer and bearable menopausal symptoms like hot flashes. The keto diet also balances blood sugar levels and insulin and helps in controlling insulin sensitivity.

Intensified Sex Drive

The keto diet surges the absorption of vitamin D, which is essential for enhancing sex drive. Vitamin D ensures stable levels of testosterone and other sex hormones that could become unstable due to low levels of testosterone.

Better Sleep

Glucose disturbs your blood sugar levels dramatically, which in turn leads to poor quality of sleep. Along with other menopausal symptoms, good sleep becomes a huge problem as you age. The keto diet for women over 50 not only balances blood glucose levels, but also stabilizes other hormones like cortisol, melatonin, and serotonin warranting an improved and better sleep.

Reduces Inflammation

Menopause can upsurge the inflammation levels by letting potential harmful invaders in our system, which result in uncomfortable and painful symptoms. Keto diet for women over 50 uses the healthy anti-inflammatory fats to reduce inflammation and lower pain in your joints and bones.

Fuel Your Brain

Are you aware that your brain is composed of 60% fat or more? This infers that it needs a larger amount of fat to keep it functioning optimally. In other words, the ketones from the keto diet serve as the energy source that fuels your brain cells.

Nutrient Deficiencies

Ageing women tend to have higher deficiencies in essential nutrients such as, iron deficiency which leads to brain fog and fatigue; Vitamin B12 deficiency, which leads to neurological conditions like dementia; Fats deficiency, that can lead to problems with cognition, skin, vision; and Vitamin D deficiency that not only causes cognitive impairment in older adults and increase the risk of heart disease but also contribute to the risk of developing cancer. On a keto diet, the high-quality proteins ensure adequate and excellent sources of these important nutrients.

Controlling Blood Sugar

Research has suggested a link between poor blood sugar levels and brain diseases such as Alzheimer's disease, Parkinson's Disease, or Dementia. Some factors contributing to Alzheimer's disease may include: - Enormous intake of carbohydrates, especially from fructose—which is drastically reduced in the ketogenic diet.

How to Start after 50?

As you get older, it gets harder for you to make decisions. But if you want to gain more energy and stay fit in your 50s, you should try the Keto diet. Below, you'll find the complete guide for beginners.

Here are some simple steps that'll help you start the low-carb diet successfully:

Reduce Your Carb Intake to 20 Grams per Day

This is the crucial rule of the Keto diet because only if the carb levels are very-very low can your body produce ketones. However, this rule doesn't refer to fiber that can be highly effective in stimulating ketone levels.

Keep Moderate Protein Consumption

Here, 'moderate' means no less than 25 percent of calories. For example, if your weight is 70 kilos, you can eat about 100 grams of protein per day. You should know that consuming too much protein can stop ketosis because the body can turn excess protein into glucose.

Regulate Sleep Patterns

People over 50 should sleep 8-9 hours per night. Keep that in mind as sleep deprivation may cause slower ketosis.

Ensure You are Consuming enough Fat

The whole idea of the Keto diet is increasing your fat intake. So be sure you add enough fat to your meals to feel energized and full. Just try not to overeat and not to eat when you don't feel hungry.

Practice Intermittent Fasting

If you skip one or two meals during the day several times a week, this can also stimulate ketosis as well as speed up weight loss.

Keep Moderate Protein Consumption

Do no less than 25 percent of calories. For example, if your weight is 70 kilos, you can eat about 100 grams of protein per day. You should know that consuming too much protein can stop ketosis because the body can turn excess protein into glucose.

Try to Get in Some Exercise

Inserting any kind of physical activity when sticking to the Keto diet may also speed up ketosis. This is not a requirement. However, visiting a sports gym can have a positive effect not only on physical but also mental health.

Most Common Mistakes and How to Fix Them

Do you feel like you are giving your all to the keto diet, but you still aren't seeing the results you want? You are measuring ketones, working out, and counting your macros, but you still aren't losing the weight you want. Here are the most common mistakes that most people make when beginning the keto diet.

Too Many Snacks

There are many snacks you can enjoy while following the keto diet, like nuts, avocado, seeds, and cheese. But snacking can be an easy way to get too many calories into the diet while giving your body an easy fuel source besides stored fat. Snacks need to be only used if you frequently hunger between meals. If you aren't extremely hungry, let your body turn to your stored fat for its fuel between meals instead of dietary fat.

Not Consuming Enough Fat

The ketogenic diet isn't all about low carbs. It's also about high fats. You need to be getting about 75 percent of your calories from healthy fats, five percent from carbs, and 20 percent from protein. Fat makes you feel fuller longer, so if you eat the correct amount, you will minimize your carb cravings, and this will help you stay in ketosis. This will help your body burn fat faster.

Consuming Excessive Calories

You may hear people say you can eat what you want on the keto diet as long as it is high in fat. Even though we want that to be true, it is very misleading. Healthy fats need to make up the biggest part of your diet. If you eat more calories than what you are burning, you will gain weight, no matter what you eat because these excess calories get stored as fat. An average adult only needs about 2,000 calories each day, but this will vary based on many factors like activity level, height, and gender.

Consuming a lot of Dairies

For many people, dairy can cause inflammation and keeps them from losing weight. Dairy is a combo food meaning it has carbs, protein, and fats. If you eat a lot of cheese as a snack for the fat content, you are also getting a dose of carbs and protein with that fat. Many people can tolerate dairy, but moderation is the key. Stick with no more than one to two ounces of cheese or cream at each meal. Remember to factor in the protein content.

Consuming a lot of Protein

The biggest mistake that most people make when just beginning the keto diet is consuming too much protein. Excess protein gets converted into glucose in the body called gluconeogenesis. This is a natural process where the body converts the energy from fats and proteins into glucose when glucose isn't available. When following a ketogenic diet, gluconeogenesis happens at different rates to keep body function. Our bodies don't need a lot of carbs, but we do need glucose. You can eat absolute zero carbs, and through gluconeogenesis, your body will convert other substances into glucose to be used as fuel. This is why carbs only make up five percent of your macros. Some parts of our bodies need carbs to survive, like kidney, medulla, and red blood cells. With gluconeogenesis, our bodies make and stores extra glucose as glycogen just in case supplies become too low.

In a normal diet, when carbs are always available, gluconeogenesis happens slowly because the need for glucose is extremely low. Our body runs on glucose and will store excess protein and carbs as fat.

It does take time for our bodies to switch from using glucose to burning fats. Once you are in ketosis, your body will use fat as the main fuel source and will start to store excess protein as glycogen.

Not Getting Enough Water

Water is crucial for your body. Water is needed for all your body does, and this includes burning fat. If you don't drink enough water, it can cause your metabolism to slow down, and this can halt your weight loss. Drinking 64 ounces or one-half gallon every day will help your body burn fat, flush out toxins, and circulate nutrients. When you are just beginning the keto diet, you might need to drink more water since your body will begin to get rid of body fat by flushing it out through urine.

Consuming Too Many Sweets

Some people might indulge in keto brownies and keto cookies that are full of sugar substitute just because their net carb content is low, but you have to remember that you are still eating calories. Eating sweets might increase your carb cravings. Keto sweets are great on occasion; they don't need to be a staple in the diet.

Not Getting Enough Sleep

Getting plenty of sleep is needed in order to lose weight effectively. Without the right amount of sleep, your body will feel stressed, and this could result in your metabolism slowing down. It might cause it to store fat instead of burning fat. When you feel tired, you are more tempted to drink more lattes for energy, eat a snack to give you an extra boost, or order takeout rather than cooking a healthy meal. Try to get between seven and nine hours of sleep each night. Understand that your body uses that time to burn fat without you even lifting a finger.

Low on Electrolytes

Most people will experience the keto flu when you begin this diet. This happens for two reasons when your body changes from burning carbs to burning fat, your brain might not have enough energy, and this, in turn, can cause grogginess, headaches, and nausea. You could be dehydrated, and your electrolytes might be low since the keto diet causes you to urinate often.

Getting the keto flu is a great sign that you are heading in the right direction. You can lessen these symptoms by drinking more water or taking supplements that will balance your electrolytes.

Consuming Hidden Carbs

Many foods look like they are low carb, but they aren't. You can find carbs in salad dressings, sauces, and condiments. Be sure to check nutrition labels before you try new foods to make sure it doesn't have any hidden sugar or carbs. It just takes a few seconds to skim the label, and it might be the difference between whether or not you'll lose weight.

If you have successfully ruled out all of the above, but you still aren't losing weight, you might need to talk with your doctor to make sure you don't have any health problems that could be preventing your weight loss. This can be frustrating, but stick with it. Stay positive and stay in the game. When the keto diet is done correctly, it is one of the best ways to lose weight.

Benefits of Following Keto Diet for Women Over 50

The Keto diet has been proven to have many benefits for people over 50. Here are some of the best.

Eradicates Inflammation

Few things are worse than the pain from an inflamed joint or muscle. Arthritis, for instance, can be extremely difficult to bear. When you follow the ketosis diet, the production of cytokines will be reduced. Cytokines cause inflammation, and therefore, their eradication will reduce it.

It Eradicates Nutrients Deficiency

Keto focuses on consuming exactly what you need. If you use a great Keto plan, your body will lack no nutrients and will not suffer any deficiency.

Reduced Hunger

The reason we find it difficult to stick to diets is hunger. It doesn't matter your age; diets do not become easier. We may have a mental picture of the healthy body we want. We may even have clear visuals of the kind of life we want to lead once free from unhealthy living, but none of that matters when hunger enters the scene. However, the Keto diet is a diet that combats this problem. The Keto diet focuses on consuming plenty of proteins. Proteins are filling and do not let you feel hungry too easily. Besides, when your carb levels are reduced, your appetite takes a hit. It is a win-win situation.

Weight Loss

Keto not only burns fat, but it also reduces that craving for food. Combined, these are two great ways to lose weight. It is one of the diets that has proven to help the most when it comes to weight loss. The Keto diet has been proven to be one of the best ways to burn stubborn belly fat while keeping yourself revitalized and healthy.

Reduces Blood Sugar and Insulin

After 50, monitoring blood sugar can be a real struggle. Cutting down on carbs drastically reduces both insulin levels and blood sugar levels. This means that the Keto diet will benefit millions as many people struggle with insulin complications and high blood sugar levels. It has been proven to help as when some people embark on Keto, and they cut up to half of the carbs they consume. It's a treasure for those with diabetes and insulin resistance. A study was carried out on people with type 2 diabetes. After cutting down on carbs, within six months, 95 percent of people were able to reduce or stop using their glucose-lowering medication.

Lower Levels of Triglycerides

Many people do not know what triglycerides are. Triglycerides are molecules of fat in your blood. They are known to circulate the bloodstream and can be very dangerous. High levels of triglycerides can cause heart failures and heart diseases. However, Keto is known to reduce these levels.

Reduces Acne

Although acne is mostly suffered by those who are young, there are cases of people above 50 having it. Moreover, Keto is not only for persons after 50. Acne is not only caused by blocked pores. There are quite some things proven to cause it. One of these things is your blood sugar. When you consume processed and refined carbs, it affects gut bacteria and results in the fluctuation of blood sugar levels. When the gut bacteria and sugar levels are affected, the skin suffers. However, when you embark on the Keto diet, you cut off on carbs intake, which means that in the very first place, your gut bacteria will not be affected, thereby cutting off that avenue to develop.

Increases HDL Levels

HDL refers to high-density lipoprotein. When your HDL levels are compared to your LDL levels and are not found low, your risk of developing heart disease is lowered. This is great for persons over 50 as heart diseases suddenly become more probable. Eating fats and reducing your intake of carbohydrates is one of the most certain ways to increase your high-density lipoprotein levels.

Reduces LDL Levels

High levels of LDL can be very problematic when you attain 50. This is because LDL refers to bad cholesterol. People with high levels of this cholesterol are more likely to get heart attacks. When you reduce the number of carbs you consume, you will increase the size of bad LDL particles. However, this will result in the reduction of the total LDL particles as they would have increased in size. Smaller LDL particles have been linked to heart diseases, while larger ones have been proven to have lower risks attached.

May Help Combat Cancer

I termed this under 'may' because research on this is not as extensive and conclusive as we would like it to be. However, there is proof of supporting it. Firstly, it helps reduce the levels of blood sugar, which in turn reduces insulin complications, which in turn reduces the risk of developing cancers related to insulin levels. Besides, Keto places more oxidative stress on cancer cells than on normal cells, thereby making it great for chemotherapy. The risk of developing cancer after fifty is still existent, and so, Keto is a lifesaver.

May Lower Blood Pressure

High blood pressure plagues adults much more than it does young ones. Once you attain 50, you must monitor your blood pressure rates. Reduction in the intake of carbohydrates is a proven way to lower your blood pressure. When you cut down on your carbs and lower your blood sugar levels, you greatly reduce your chances of getting some other diseases.

Combats Metabolic Syndrome

As you grow older, you may find that you struggle to control your blood sugar level. Metabolic syndrome is another condition that has been proven to influence diabetes and heart disease development. The symptoms associated with metabolic syndrome include but are not limited to high triglycerides, obesity, high blood sugar level, and low levels of high-density lipoprotein cholesterol.

Great for the Heart

People over the age of 50 have been proven to have more chances of developing heart diseases. Keto diet has been proven to be great for the heart. As it increases good cholesterol levels and reduces the levels of bad cholesterol, you will find that partaking in the Keto diet proves extremely beneficial for your health.

May Reduce Seizure Risks

When you change your intake levels, the combination of protein, fat, and carbs, as we explained before, your body will go into ketosis. Ketosis has been proven to reduce seizure levels in people who have epilepsy. When they do not respond to treatment, the ketosis treatment is used. This has been done for decades.

Combats Brain Disorders

Keto doesn't end there, and it also combats Alzheimer's and Parkinson's disease. Some parts of your brain can only burn glucose, and so, your body needs it. If you do not consume carbs, your lover will make use of protein to produce glucose. Your brain can also burn ketones. Ketones are formed when your carb level is very low.

Bone Health

Osteoporosis becomes more likely as a person advances in age. This is especially true if you weren't able to introduce appropriate amounts of calcium in your body. As you probably know, osteoporosis makes the bone brittle and fragile. This means that your likelihood of having serious injury from seemingly small accidents increases. A simple slip and bones can fracture, or hips may become dislocated. Persistent inflammation of the joints could become an everyday problem. The Ketogenic Diet is a good way of preventing these from happening because the diet naturally involves the intake of healthy dairy or milk products. More importantly, the Ketogenic Diet promotes the intake of low-toxin food products.

CHAPTER 3:

Intermittent Fasting and Keto Diet

What is Intermittent Fasting Diet?

Intermittent fasting (IF) is when a person refrains from eating during certain hours of the day. During the hours that the person is not fasting, they eat a healthy, regimented diet. The intermittent fasting diet is not so much of a diet but a lifestyle change.

Some of the more popular intermittent fasting methods are two to three days a week, alternate days, or daily during set hours. The thing about the intermittent fasting diet is that there is no need for counting calories, macronutrients, or cutting down on certain foods.

There are no set rules other than not eating certain set rules, and you can eat what you like during the time window in which you are not fasting. During the time when you are fasting, you can drink water, tea, and coffee.

Intermittent fasting is a diet that can be used to lose weight, enhance body composition, and decrease body fat. It has been known to have a lot of other health benefits, especially for women in middle age.

Why for Women Over 50?

Women who approach post-menopause (and sometimes even as early as pre-menopause) tend to start accumulating belly fat. They will start noticing their metabolism get slower. They may also start feeling aches and pains in their joints. Their sleep patterns start to get completely out of routine leaving them feeling exhausted all the time. Then there is the weight gain and also a higher risk of developing chronic diseases like cancer, diabetes, and heart disease that could lead to heart attacks.

There is also the risk of neurodegenerative diseases, stroke, and a constant feeling of fatigue. Intermittent fasting has been known to reset a person's internal balance. This, in turn, boosts their external appearance, energy levels, and cuts down on stress as they control their weight.

Intermittent fasting has become a very popular healthy lifestyle trend, and for good reason. It offers many health benefits as well as improves a person's state of mind and encourages an all-round feeling of wellbeing.

Benefits of Intermittent Fasting for Women Over 50

When women get to 50 and over, their skin will start to show signs of age. They may find their joints start to ache for no reason, and suddenly belly fat accumulates as if you have just given birth. There are so many creams, diets, and exercises on the market to tighten the skin and try to help. The fact is, they may work to a certain point but then the body hits a shelf, and nothing seems to push a person past it. This boils up frustration making women look into the more drastic and very expensive alternatives like surgery. Which in itself poses so many more dangers and risks for women of 50 and over.

A person does not need to go under the knife or starve themselves to reboot their system or change their shape. Intermittent fasting is a much cheaper and less risky way to do this and there is no need to make any drastic eating habit changes either. Well, you may need to make a few adjustments like cutting out junk food and eating healthier. But once again the diet a person follows is their personal choice and depends on how serious they are about becoming healthier.

Some health benefits of intermittent fasting for women over 50 include:

Activating Cellular Repair

Fasting has been known to kick start the body's natural cellular repair function, get rid of mature cells, improve longevity, and improve hormone function. All things that tend to take a battering as people age. This can alleviate joint and muscle aches as well as lower back pain. As the cells are being repaired and damage undone, it helps with the skin's elasticity and health too.

Increase Cognitive Function and Protects the Brain from Damage

Intermittent fasting may increase the levels of a brain hormone known as a Brain-Derived Neurotrophic Factor (BDNF). It may equally guard the brain against damage like a stroke or Alzheimer's disease as it promotes new nerve cell growth. It also increases cognitive function and could effectively defend a person against other neurodegenerative diseases as well.

Weight Loss

When people have belly fat, it can cause many health problems that are associated with various diseases as it indicates a person has visceral fat. Visceral fat is fat that goes deep into the abdominal surrounding the organs. Belly fat is terribly hard to lose, especially for an aging woman. Intermittent fasting has been known to help reduce not only weight but inches of over five percent of body fat in around twenty-two to twenty-five weeks (Barna, 2019).

Alleviates Oxidative Stress and Inflammation

Intermittent fasting can provide your system with a reboot, helping to alleviate oxidative stress and inflammation in a middle-aged woman. It also significantly reduces the risk of oxidative stress and inflammation for those overweight or obese.

Slow Down the Aging Process

As intermittent fasting gives both the metabolism and cellular repair a reboot. It offers the potential to slow down aging. It may even prolong a person's lifespan by quite a few years especially if following a nutritious diet and exercise regime alongside intermittent fasting.

Keto Diet & Intermittent Fasting

If you did some research before the keto diet, then you're probably aware of intermittent fasting. This is more or less just a fancy of way of saying that there will be a gap between fasting and eating. But the real question is, should you be doing intermittent fasting and keto at the same time? Is it healthy? Well, before we dive into these questions, let's cover the basics first.

Before you try to strike a balance between the two, perhaps it's best that you understand how each lifestyle change works on its own.

As for keto, we've already talked about how the diet is about cutting down carbs. The ultimate goal of the keto diet is to reach ketosis, enabling the body to utilize ketones for energy instead of glucose. On the other hand, intermittent fasting is more about going without food for certain hours during the day. The most popular method involves fasting for 16 hours and then having an eating window of eight hours. Rest assured, those 16 hours can also cover your bedtime so it's not like you're starving yourself.

The most popular kind of fasts includes:

12-Hour Fasting Period

As long as you're fasting, why not go half and half? Most folks find the 12-12 routine pretty easy. You can either skip the evening snacks or go the day without breakfast which should take care of your fasting and eating window.

16-Hour Fasting Period

You basically fast for 16 hours and then have an eating window of eight hours.

5:2 Method

If a 16-hour fasting window is too long for you, break it down and opt for the 5:2 method. This approach requires a caloric restriction for two days in a week followed by a regular diet for rest of the five days. For women, the caloric intake should not be more than 500 calories on the day of the fast, while for men the limit is 600 calories. Since there are no fasting days for five days a week, it is easier for seniors to follow.

Fasting Alternative Days

Another simple variation is to simply fast every other day. When and how to initiate the fast and for how many hours depends on personal preference.

First off, it's important to keep in mind that keto and intermittent fasting offer similar benefits, this includes faster metabolism, weight loss, and so on. Keeping this in mind following both diets at the same time can offer additional benefits.

For instance, like keto, fasting too encourages the body to use up fat for energy. Hence when combined with keto can help the body reach the state of ketosis more quickly. Studies have also shown how the two can result in higher fat loss levels along with increased energy levels. Seniors can combine the two if they're looking to lose some weight in the process too.

All in all, we do recommend you visit your doctor before you make any drastic dietary changes to your diet. Also, people who are not used to fasting may experience weakness, loss of energy or even fainting. Hence, in the beginning, it's a good idea to fast for shorter periods of time to allow your body to get accustomed to these new changes.

How Intermittent Fasting Can Help Stimulate Autophagy

Remember how we talked about autophagy in the earlier chapters? The phenomenon basically translates to self-eating at cellular level. This is basically the body's way of getting rid of dead cells.

Fasting is among the most effective ways to stimulate this process. It reduces glucose levels which induces a number of beneficial metabolic changes that can help your body. Autophagy helps clear out old, worn out cells and protein junk from the system. At the same, intermittent fasting also activates growth hormones that start replacing old cells. This repair and recycling processes are very helpful for the body.

Possible Side Effects of Intermittent Fasting

Before you completely take the plunge, it's important that you're aware of the possible side effects of intermittent fasting. Here are some common symptoms that you need to be aware of:

Hunger

Well, this one is pretty obvious, and it's bound to occur if you're already on a low-carb diet. We do suggest you consume nutritious food during your eating window to prevent you from feeling hungry during your fast.

Headaches

Rest assured, headaches are common side effects and tend to go after a while. Consuming some extra salt during your eating window may ease some of the chances of unpleasantness.

Constipation

Since your body is consuming fewer calories, constipation may become a problem. Keep in mind that this is normal response to eating less. You don't have to worry too much uncles you experience excessive bloating or abdominal discomfort. You can consume magnesium supplements or over-the-counter laxatives to feel better.

Refeeding Syndrome

This is a serious and almost fatal side effect after a starvation or malnourishment experience. Fortunately, it only occurs if you fast for 5-10 days.

Other common side effects include heart burn, muscle cramps and dizziness. But these side effects aren't anything major and tend to go away once you've had something to eat.

Safe Fasting Tips for Women Over 50

Fasting is a drastic life change, especially if this is something you've never tried before. Here are a couple of tips that will help you safely fast during your keto adventure:

Eating Wholesome Food

Add wholefoods to your diet, during your non-fasting periods obviously. Since the whole point of fasting along with keto is to improve your health, we highly suggest you start making some additional healthy changes to your lifestyle.

Consume Supplements

If you're serious about fasting and starting keto, you'll likely need to add supplements to your diet. This makes sense because consuming fewer calories means that it'll be more difficult for you to consume your daily dose of nutrition. Most people who opt for weight loss are generally deficient in essential nutrients such as vitamin B12, calcium and iron. However, you can also consult your physician for a more thorough analysis of what supplements you should be taking.

Replenish Fluids & Stay Hydrated

Not staying hydrated or mild dehydration can easily lead to symptoms such as headaches, dry mouth, and fatigue. We recommend your stick to the old good fashioned rule of drinking eight glasses of water and this roughly translates to about two liters.

Listen to Your Body

And of course, listen to your body. If you're feeling weak and frail, don't hesitate to break your fast. In case of any severe side effects, you should also visit your physician.

While these guidelines will take care of most of your doubts and questions, go with your instincts and figure out what works best for you.

Realize That Fasting Isn't Necessary for All

Understand that fasting isn't necessary for everybody. Here are some people who should particularly be cautious of fasting: folks who are suffering from a medical condition, especially something severe such heart disease.

Seniors who experience low blood pressure and who are on prescription medicines should also get in touch with a doctor just to be sure. Same applies for people who are already underweight and have been advised against fasting.

Fasting Doesn't Mean You Can Spend Time Feasting

Don't starve yourself but don't use fasting as an excuse to enjoy a major feast afterwards.

Consuming an incredibly calorie-rich meal can have you feeling tired and bloated afterwards.

Also, if one of your major goals is to lose weight, feasting afterwards may just disrupt your chances of that. The best way to handle the situation is to eat as you normally would (abiding to keto guidelines) once you have finished your fasting period.

CHAPTER 4:

Keto Recipes 200

BREAKFAST

Cheesy Sausage Quiche

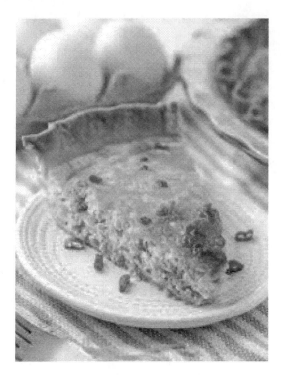

Preparation time: 5 minutes

Cooking time: 40 minutes

Servings: 4

Ingredients

- 6 eggs

- 12 ounces raw sausage roll

- 10 cherry tomatoes, halved

- 2 tbsp heavy cream

- 2 tbsp Parmesan cheese

- ¼ tsp salt

- A pinch of black pepper

- 2 tbsp chopped parsley

- 5 eggplant slices

Directions

1. Preheat your oven to 370°F.

2. Grease a pie dish with cooking spray. Press the sausage roll at the bottom of a pie dish. Arrange the eggplant slices on top of the sausage. Top with cherry tomatoes.

3. Whisk the eggs along with the heavy cream, salt, Parmesan cheese, and black pepper. Spoon the mixture over the sausage. Bake for about 40 minutes until browned around the edges. Serve warm, sprinkled with parsley.

Nutrition:

- Calories: 504;

- Carbohydrates: 33.8g;

- Protein: 7.6g;

- Fat: 39.9g;

- Sugar: 5.6g;

- Sodium: 47mg

Coconut Porridge

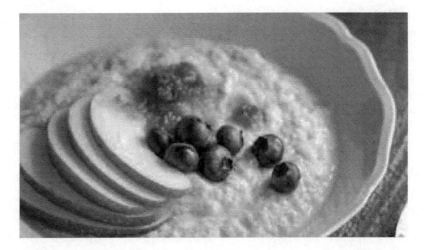

Preparation time: 5 minutes

Cooking time: 30 minutes

Servings: 4

Ingredients:

- ¼ cup unsweetened coconut flakes

- 1 tbsp. coconut flour

- 1/3 cup unsweetened coconut milk

- 1-2 tsp. monk fruit sweetener

- ¼ cup hemp seeds

- ½ cup water

- 1 tsp. organic vanilla extract

Directions:

In a pan, add the coconut, hemp seeds, water and coconut milk over medium heat and bring to boil, stirring frequently. Simmer for about 2 minutes, stirring continuously. Stir in the vanilla extract and sweetener and remove from the heat. Serve with your desired topping.

Nutrition: Calories: 226; Carbohydrates: 37.1g; Protein: 4.6g; Fat: 7.9g; Sugar: 4g; Sodium: 239mg

Bacon Omelet

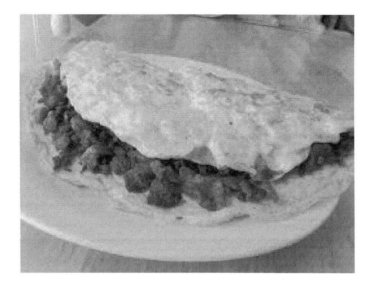

Preparation Time: 10 minutes
Cooking Time: 15 minutes
Servings: 3

Ingredients

- 4 large organic eggs

- 1 tablespoon fresh chives, minced

- Salt and ground black pepper, as required

- 4 bacon slices

- 1 tablespoon unsalted butter

- 2 ounces cheddar cheese, shredded

Directions

1. In a bowl, add the eggs, chives, salt, and black pepper, and beat until well combined.

2. Heat a nonstick frying pan over medium-high heat and cook the bacon slices for about 8–10 minutes.

3. Place the bacon onto a paper towel-lined plate to drain. Then chop the bacon slices.

4. With paper towels, wipe out the frying pan.

5. In the same frying pan, melt butter over medium-low heat and cook the egg mixture for about 2 minutes.

6. Carefully, flip the omelet and top with chopped bacon.

7. Cook for 1–2 minutes or until desired doneness of eggs.

8. Remove from heat and immediately, place the cheese in the center of omelet.

9. Fold the edges of omelet over cheese and cut into 2 portions.

10. Serve immediately.

Nutrition: Calories: 366; Carbohydrates: 44.8g; Protein: 5.8g; Fat: 18.6g; Sugar: 2.4g; Sodium: 106mg

Green Veggies Quiche

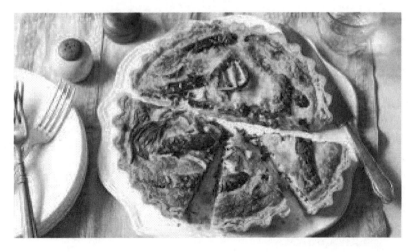

Preparation Time: 20 minutes
Cooking Time: 20 minutes
Servings: 5

Ingredients

- 6 organic eggs

- ½ cup unsweetened almond milk

- Salt and ground black pepper, as required

- 2 cups fresh baby spinach, chopped

- ½ cup green bell pepper, seeded and chopped 1 scallion, chopped

- ¼ cup fresh cilantro, chopped

- 1 tablespoon fresh chives, minced

- 3 tablespoons mozzarella cheese, grated

Directions

1. Preheat your oven to 400°F.

2. Lightly grease a pie dish.

3. In a bowl, add eggs, almond milk, salt, and black pepper, and beat until well combined. Set aside.

4. In another bowl, add the vegetables and herbs and mix well.

5. In the bottom of the prepared pie dish, place the veggie mixture evenly and top with the egg mixture.

6. Bake for about 20 minutes or until a wooden skewer inserted in the center comes out clean.

7. Remove the pie dish from the oven and immediately sprinkle with the Parmesan cheese.

8. Set aside for about 5 minutes before slicing.

9. Cut into desired sized wedges and serve warm.

Nutrition:

- Calories 618

- Fat: 47.2g,

- Carbohydrates: 31.2g,

- Dietary Fiber: 11.8g,

- Protein: 17.3g

Chicken & Asparagus Frittata

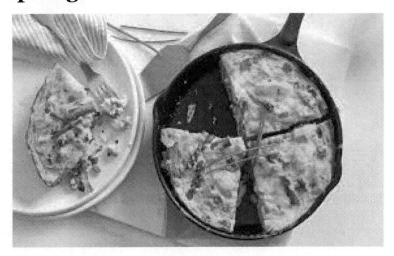

Preparation Time: 15 minutes
Cooking Time: 12 minutes
Servings: 4

Ingredients

- ½ cup grass-fed cooked chicken breast, chopped

- 1/3 cup Parmesan cheese, grated

- 6 organic eggs, beaten lightly

- Salt and ground black pepper, as required

- 1/3 cup boiled asparagus, chopped

- ¼ cup cherry tomatoes halved

- ¼ cup mozzarella cheese, shredded

Directions

1. Preheat the broiler of the oven.

2. In a bowl, add the Parmesan cheese, eggs, salt, and black pepper, and beat until well combined.

3. In a large ovenproof wok, melt butter over medium-high heat and cook the chicken and asparagus for about 2–3 minutes.

4. Add the egg mixture and tomatoes and stir to combine.

5. Cook for about 4–5 minutes.

6. Remove from the heat and sprinkle with the Parmesan cheese.

7. Now, transfer the wok under the broiler and broil for about 3–4 minutes or until slightly puffed.

8. Cut into desired sized wedges and serve immediately.

Nutrition:

- Calorie: 187

- Carbohydrates: 25.9g

- Protein: 4.5g

- Fat: 7.2g

- Sugar: 10.6g

- Sodium: 303mg

Ricotta Cloud Pancakes with Whipped Cream

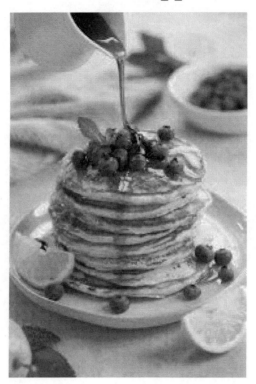

Preparation time: 5 minutes

Cooking time: 30 minutes

Servings: 4

Ingredients

- 1 cup almond flour

- 1 tsp baking powder

- 2 ½ tbsp swerve

- ⅓ tsp salt

- 1 ¼ cups ricotta cheese

- ⅓ cup coconut milk

- 2 large eggs

- 1 cup heavy whipping cream

Directions

1. In a medium bowl, whisk the almond flour, baking powder, swerve, and salt. Set aside.

2. Crack the eggs into the blender and process on medium speed for 30 seconds. Add the ricotta cheese, continue processing it, and gradually pour the coconut milk in while you keep on blending. In about 90 seconds, the mixture will be creamy and smooth. Pour it into the dry ingredients and whisk to combine.

3. Set a skillet over medium heat and let it heat for a minute. Then, fetch a soup spoonful of mixture into the skillet and cook it for 1 minute.

4. Flip the pancake and cook further for 1 minute. Remove onto a plate and repeat the cooking process until the batter is exhausted. Serve the pancakes with whipping cream.

Nutrition:

- Calories 253
- Fat: 11.03g
- Carbohydrates 0.93g
- Fiber 0.17g
- Protein 34.95g

Mushroom & Cheese Lettuce Wraps

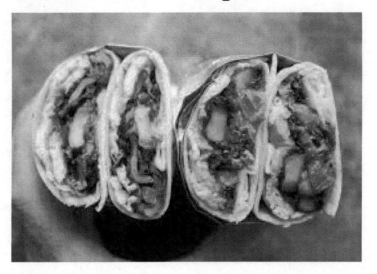

Preparation time: 5 minutes

Cooking time: 20 minutes

Servings: 4

Ingredients

For the Wraps:

- 6 eggs

- 2 tbsp almond milk

- 1 tbsp olive oil

- Sea salt, to taste

- For the Filling:

- 1 tsp olive oil

- 1 cup mushrooms, chopped

- Salt and black pepper, to taste

- ½ tsp cayenne pepper

- 8 fresh lettuce leaves

- 4 slices gruyere cheese

- 2 tomatoes, sliced

Directions

1. Mix all the ingredients for the wraps thoroughly.

2. Set a frying pan over medium heat. Add in ¼ of the mixture and cook for 4 minutes on both sides. Do the same thrice and set the wraps aside, they should be kept warm.

3. In a separate pan over medium heat, warm 1 teaspoon of olive oil. Cook the mushrooms for 5 minutes until soft; add cayenne pepper, black pepper, and salt.

4. Set 1-2 lettuce leaves onto every wrap, split the mushrooms among the wraps and top with tomatoes and cheese.

Nutrition:

- Calories 349,23

- Fat:28.77g

- Carbohydrates 5,27g

- Fiber 0,72g

- Protein 18,61g

Bacon & Cheese Pesto Mug Cakes

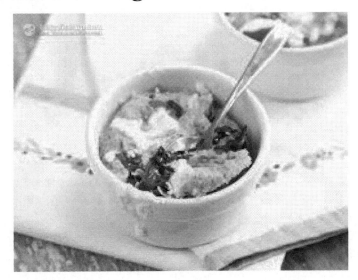

Preparation time: 5 minutes

Cooking time: 30 minutes

Servings: 4

Ingredients

- ¼ cup flax meal

- 1 egg

- 2 tbsp heavy cream

- 2 tbsp pesto

- ¼ cup almond flour

- ¼ tsp baking soda

- Salt and black pepper, to taste

Filling:

- 2 tbsp cream cheese

- 4 slices bacon

- ½ medium avocado, sliced

Directions

1. Mix together the dry muffin ingredients in a bowl. Add egg, heavy cream, and pesto, and whisk well with a fork. Season with salt and pepper. Divide the mixture between two ramekins.

2. Place in the microwave and cook for 60-90 seconds. Leave to cool slightly before filling.

3. Meanwhile, in a skillet, over medium heat, cook the bacon slices until crispy. Transfer to paper towels to soak up excess fat; set aside. Invert the muffins onto a plate and cut in half, crosswise.

4. To assemble the sandwiches: spread cream cheese and top with bacon and avocado slices.

Nutrition:

- Calories 161
- Fat: 12.05
- Carbohydrates 4.97g
- Fiber: 3.24g
- Protein 9,35g

Mascarpone & Vanilla Breakfast Cups

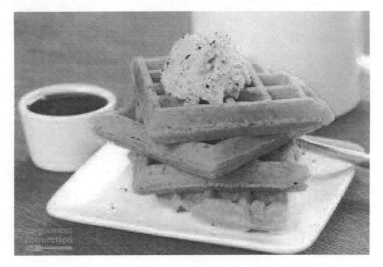

Preparation time: 5 minutes

Cooking time: 40 minutes

Servings: 4

Ingredients

- ¾ cup mascarpone cheese

- ¼ cup natural yogurt

- 3 eggs, beaten

- 1 tbsp walnuts, ground

- 4 tbsp erythritol

- ½ tsp vanilla essence

- ⅓ tsp ground cinnamon

Directions

1. Set oven to 360°F and grease a muffin pan. Mix all ingredients in a bowl. Split the batter into the muffin cups.

2. Bake for 12 to 15 minutes. Remove and set on a wire rack to cool slightly before serving.

Nutrition:

- Calories 216

- Fat 2.9 g

- Carbohydrates 43.9 g

- Sugar 12.1 g

- Protein 5.7 g

- Cholesterol 0 mg

Quickly Blue Cheese Omelet

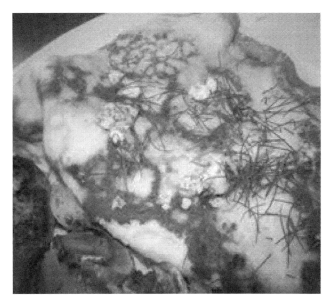

Preparation time: 5 minutes

Cooking time: 50 minutes

Servings: 4

Ingredients

- 4 eggs

- Salt, to taste

- 1 tbsp sesame oil

- ½ cup blue cheese, crumbled

- 1 tomato, thinly sliced

Directions

1. In a mixing bowl, beat the eggs and season with salt.

2. Set a sauté pan over medium heat and warm the oil. Add in the eggs and cook as you swirl the eggs around the pan using a spatula. Cook eggs until partially set.

3. Top with cheese; fold the omelet in half to enclose filling. Decorate with tomato and serve while warm.

Nutrition

- Calories –248

- Fat – 5.5g

- Carbohydrates – 52g

- Fiber – 13g

- Protein – 7g

Breakfast Buttered Eggs

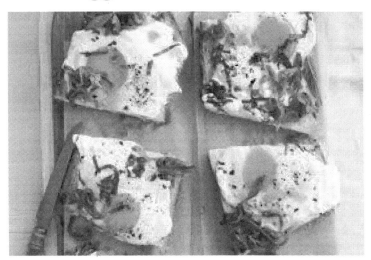

Preparation time: 5 minutes

Cooking time: 30 minutes

Servings: 4

Ingredients

- 1 tbsp coconut oil
- 2 tbsp butter
- 1 tsp fresh thyme
- 4 eggs
- 2 garlic cloves, minced
- ½ cup chopped parsley
- ½ cup chopped cilantro
- ¼ tsp cumin
- ¼ tsp cayenne pepper
- Salt and black pepper, to taste

Directions

1. Drizzle the coconut oil into a nonstick skillet over medium heat. Once the oil is warm, add the butter, and melt.

2. Add garlic and thyme and cook for 30 seconds. Sprinkle with parsley and cilantro; and cook for another 2 minutes, until crisp.

3. Carefully crack the eggs into the skillet. Lower the heat and cook for 4-6 minutes. Season with salt, black pepper, cumin, and cayenne pepper.

4. When the eggs are just set, turn the heat off and transfer to a serving plate.

Nutrition:

- Calories: 244

- Carbohydrates: 27.8g

- Protein: 3.2g

- Fat: 14.3g

- Sugar: 2.4g

- Sodium: 670mg

Bacon & Cheese Zucchini Balls

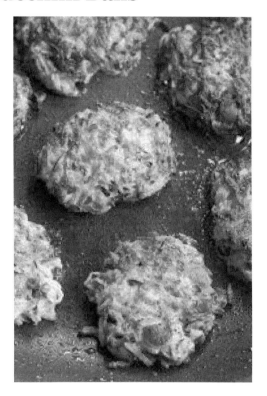

Preparation time: 5 minutes

Cooking time: 30 minutes

Servings: 4

Ingredients

- 4 cups zoodles

- ½ pound bacon, chopped

- 6 ounces cottage cheese, curds

- 6 ounces cream cheese

- 1 cup fontina cheese

- ½ cup dill pickles, chopped, squeezed

- 2 cloves garlic, crushed

- 1 cup grated Parmesan cheese

- ½ tsp caraway seeds

- ¼ tsp dried dill weed

- ½ tsp onion powder

- Salt and black pepper, to taste

- 1 cup crushed pork rinds

- Cooking oil

Directions

1. Thoroughly mix zoodles, cottage cheese, dill pickles, ½ cup of Parmesan cheese, garlic, cream cheese, bacon, and fontina cheese until well combined. Shape the mixture into balls. Refrigerate for 3 hours.

2. In a mixing bowl, mix the remaining ½ cup of Parmesan cheese, crushed pork rinds, dill, black pepper, onion powder, caraway seeds, and salt. Roll cheese ball in Parmesan mixture to coat.

3. Set a skillet over medium heat and warm 1-inch of oil. Fry cheeseballs until browned on all sides. Set on a paper towel to soak up any excess oil.

Nutrition:

- Calories: 122

- Carbohydrates: 11.5g

- Protein: 5.1g

- Fat: 8g

- Sugar: 2.8g

- Sodium: 69mg

Chorizo and Mozzarella Omelet

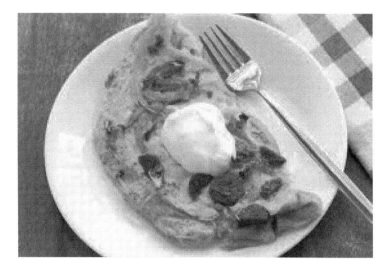

Preparation time: 5 minutes

Cooking time: 60 minutes

Servings: 4

Ingredients

- 2 eggs

- 6 basil leaves

- 2 ounces mozzarella cheese

- 1 tbsp butter

- 1 tbsp water

- 4 thin slices chorizo

- 1 tomato, sliced

- Salt and black pepper, to taste

Directions

1. Whisk the eggs along with the water and some salt and pepper. Melt the butter in a skillet and cook the eggs for 30 seconds.

2. Spread the chorizo slices over. Arrange the tomato and mozzarella over the chorizo. Cook for about 3 minutes. Cover the skillet and cook for 3 minutes until omelet is set.

3. When ready, remove the pan from heat; run a spatula around the edges of the omelet and flip it onto a warm plate, folded side down.

4. Serve garnished with basil leaves and green salad.

Nutrition:

- Calories: 571
- Carbohydrates: 45.6g
- Protein: 8.5g
- Fat: 44g
- Sugar: 15.8g
- Sodium: 32mg

Hashed Zucchini & Bacon Breakfast

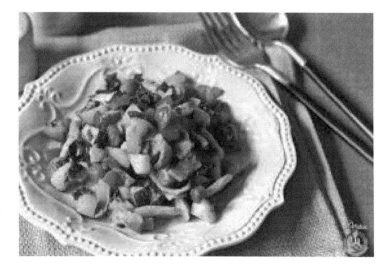

Preparation time: 5 minutes

Cooking time: 30 minutes

Servings: 4

Ingredients

- 1 medium zucchini, diced

- 2 bacon slices

- 1 egg

- 1 tbsp coconut oil

- ½ small onion, chopped

- 1 tbsp chopped parsley

- ¼ tsp salt

Directions

1. Place the bacon in a skillet and cook for a few minutes, until crispy. Remove and set aside.

2. Warm the coconut oil and cook the onion until soft, for about 3-4 minutes, occasionally stirring. Add the zucchini and cook for 10 more minutes until zucchini is brown and tender, but not mushy. Transfer to a plate and season with salt.

3. Crack the egg into the same skillet and fry over medium heat. Top the zucchini mixture with the bacon slices and a fried egg. Serve hot, sprinkled with parsley.

Nutrition:

- Calories 293

- Fat: 20.9g

- Carbohydrates: 3.2g

- Dietary Fiber: 1.3

- Protein: 23.3g

Morning Almond Shake

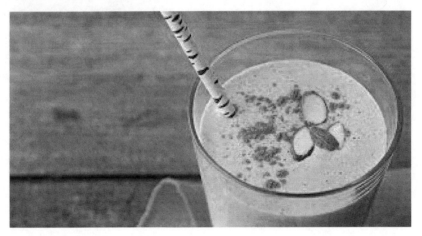

Preparation time: 5 minutes

Cooking time: 40 minutes

Servings: 4

Ingredients

- 1 ½ cups almond milk

- 2 tbsp almond butter

- ½ tsp almond extract

- ½ tsp cinnamon

- 2 tbsp flax meal

- 1 tbsp collagen peptides

- A pinch of salt

- 15 drops of stevia

- A handful of ice cubes

Directions

1. Add almond milk, almond butter, flax meal, almond extract, collagen peptides, a pinch of salt, and stevia to the bowl of a blender. Blitz until uniform and smooth, for about 30 seconds.

2. Add a bit more almond milk if it's very thick.

3. Then taste, and adjust flavor as needed, adding more stevia for sweetness or almond butter to the creaminess.

4. Pour in a smoothie glass, add the ice cubes and sprinkle with cinnamon.

Nutrition:

- Calories 235

- Fat 11 g

- Carbohydrates 31.8 g

- Sugar 21.6 g

- Protein 4.7 g

- Cholesterol 14 mg

Egg Omelet Roll with Cream Cheese & Salmon

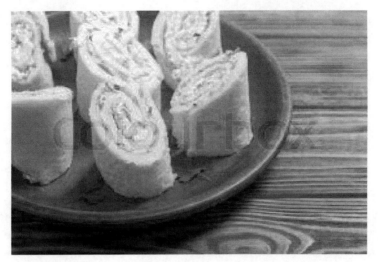

Preparation time: 5 minutes

Cooking time: 20 minutes

Servings: 4

Ingredients

- ½ avocado, sliced

- 2 tbsp chopped chives

- ½ package smoked salmon, cut into strips

- 1 spring onions, sliced

- 3 eggs

- 2 tbsp cream cheese

- 1 tbsp butter

- Salt and black pepper, to taste

Directions

1. In a small bowl, combine the chives and cream cheese; set aside. Beat the eggs in a large bowl and season with salt and black pepper.

2. Melt the butter in a pan over medium heat. Add the eggs to the pan and cook for about 3 minutes. Flip the omelet over and continue cooking for another 2 minutes until golden.

3. Remove the omelet to a plate and spread the chive mixture over. Arrange the salmon, avocado, and onion slices. Wrap the omelet and serve immediately.

Nutrition:

- Calories 403
- Fat 36.9 g
- Carbohydrates 20.4 g
- Sugar 14 g
- Protein 4.2 g
- Cholesterol 0 mg

Traditional Spinach and Feta Frittata

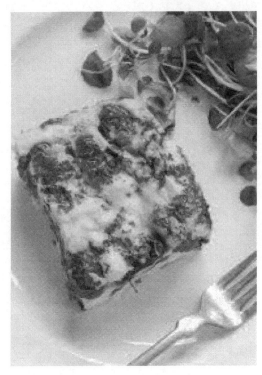

Preparation time: 5 minutes

Cooking time: 30 minutes

Servings: 4

Ingredients

- 5 ounces spinach

- 8 ounces crumbled feta cheese

- 1-pint halved cherry tomatoes

- 10 eggs

- 3 tbsp olive oil

- 4 scallions, diced

- Salt and black pepper, to taste

Directions

1. Preheat your oven to 350ºF.

2. Drizzle the oil in a casserole and place in the oven until heated. In a bowl, whisk the eggs along with the black pepper and salt, until thoroughly combined. Stir in the spinach, feta cheese, and scallions.

3. Pour the mixture into the casserole, top with the cherry tomatoes and place back in the oven. Bake for 25 minutes until your frittata is set in the middle.

4. When done, remove the casserole from the oven and run a spatula around the edges of the frittata; slide it onto a warm platter. Cut the frittata into wedges and serve with salad.

Nutrition:

- Calories 428

- Fat 17.9 g

- Carbohydrates 59.4 g

- Sugar 19.2 g

- Protein 9.9 g

- Cholesterol 0 mg

Chocolate Protein Coconut Shake

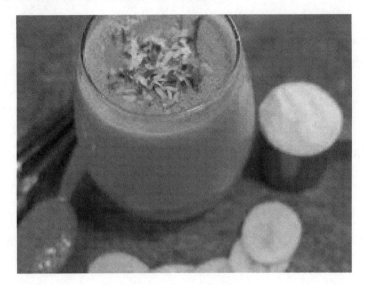

Preparation time: 5 minutes

Cooking time: 20 minutes

Servings: 4

Ingredients

- 3 cups flax milk, chilled

- 3 tsp unsweetened cocoa powder

- 1 medium avocado, pitted, peeled, sliced

- 1 cup coconut milk, chilled

- 3 mint leaves + extra to garnish

- 3 tbsp erythritol

- 1 tbsp low carb Protein powder

- Whipping cream for topping

Directions

1. Combine the flax milk, cocoa powder, avocado, coconut milk, 3 mint leaves, erythritol, and protein powder into the smoothie maker, and blend for 1 minute to smooth.

2. Pour the drink into serving glasses, lightly add some whipping cream on top, and garnish with 1 or 2 mint leaves. Serve immediately.

Nutrition:

- Calories 223

- Fat 8.8 g

- Carbohydrates 30.1 g

- Sugar 12.3 g

- Protein 7 g

- Cholesterol 8 mg

Broccoli & Colby Cheese Frittata

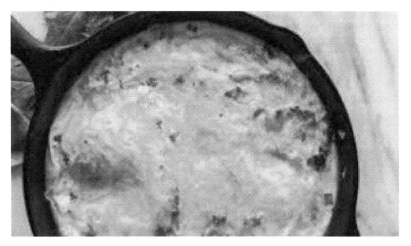

Preparation time: 5 minutes

Cooking time: 40 minutes

Servings: 4

Ingredients

- 2 tbsp olive oil

- ½ cup onions, chopped

- 1 cup broccoli, chopped

- 8 eggs, beaten

- ½ tsp jalapeño pepper, minced

- Salt and red pepper, to taste

- ¾ cup Colby cheese, grated

- ¼ cup fresh cilantro, to serve

Directions

1. Set an ovenproof frying pan over medium heat and warm the oil. Add onions and sauté until caramelized. Place in the broccoli and cook until tender. Add in jalapeno pepper and eggs; season with red pepper and salt.

2. Cook until the eggs are set.

3. Scatter Colby cheese over the frittata. Set oven to 370°F and cook for approximately 12 minutes, until frittata is set in the middle.

4. Slice into wedges and decorate with fresh cilantro before serving.

Nutrition:

- Calories 266

- Total Fats 12g

- Carbs: 31g

- Protein 9g

- Dietary Fiber: 3g

Baked Eggs in Avocados

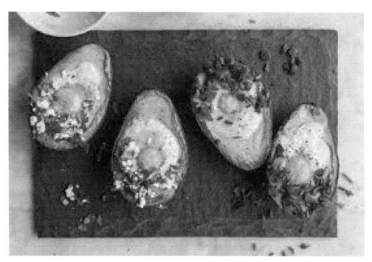

Preparation time: 5 minutes

Cooking time: 20 minutes

Servings: 4

Ingredients

- 2 large avocados, halved and pitted

- 4 small eggs

- Salt and black pepper to season

- Chopped parsley to garnish

Directions

1. Preheat the oven to 400°F.

2. Crack each egg into each avocado half and place them on a greased baking sheet. Bake the filled avocados in the oven for 8 or 10 minutes or until eggs are cooked.

3. Season with salt and pepper, and garnish with parsley.

Nutrition: Calories 372 - Total Fats 2.5g - Carbs: 35.7g - Protein 6g - Dietary Fiber: 3g

Ham and Vegetable Frittata

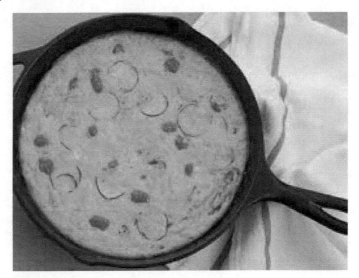

Preparation time: 5 minutes

Cooking time: 40 minutes

Servings: 4

Ingredients

- 2 tbsp butter, at room temperature

- ½ cup green onions, chopped

- 2 garlic cloves, minced

- 1 jalapeño pepper, chopped

- 1 carrot, chopped

- 8 ham slices

- 8 eggs, whisked

- Salt and black pepper, to taste

- ½ tsp dried thyme

Directions

1. Set a pan over medium heat and warm the butter. Stir in green onions and sauté for 4 minutes.

2. Place in garlic and cook for 1 minute. Stir in carrot and jalapeño pepper and cook for 4 more minutes. Remove the mixture to a lightly greased baking pan, with cooking spray, and top with ham slices.

3. Place in the eggs over vegetables and ham; add thyme, black pepper, and salt for seasoning. Bake in the oven for about 18 minutes at 360°F. Serve warm alongside a dollop of full-fat natural yogurt.

Nutrition:

- Calories 202
- Total Fats 11.6g
- Carbs: 14g
- Protein 11g
- Dietary Fiber: 2g

Eggs & Crabmeat with Creme Fraiche Salsa

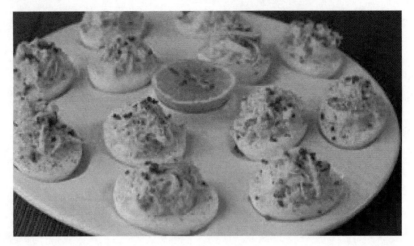

Preparation time: 5 minutes

Cooking time: 20 minutes

Servings: 4

Ingredients

- 1 tbsp olive oil

- 6 eggs, whisked

- 1 (6 oz) can crabmeat, flaked

- Salt and black pepper to taste

- For the Salsa:

- ¾ cup crème fraiche

- ½ cup scallions, chopped

- ½ tsp garlic powder

- Salt and black pepper to taste

- ½ tsp fresh dill, chopped

Directions

1. Set a sauté pan over medium heat and warm olive oil. Crack in eggs and scramble them.

2. Stir in crabmeat and season with salt and black pepper Cooking until cooked thoroughly.

3. In a mixing dish, combine all salsa ingredients.

4. Equally, split the egg/crabmeat mixture among serving plates; serve alongside the scallions and salsa to the side.

Nutrition:

- Calories 660

- Total Fats 40g

- Carbs: 8g

- Protein 40g

- Dietary Fiber: 0.3g

LUNCH

Winter Cabbage and Celery Soup

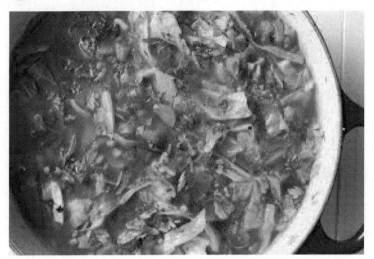

Preparation Time: 5 minutes

Cooking Time:30 minutes

Servings: 6

Ingredients:

- Tablespoon olive oil

- 2 cloves garlic, minced

- 1/2 head cabbage, shredded

- 2 stalks celery, chopped

- 1 grated tomato

- 3 cups bone broth preferable homemade

- 2 cups water

- 1/2 teaspoon ground black pepper

Directions:

1. Heat the oil in a large pot over medium heat.

2. Sauté the garlic, celery and cabbage, stirring, for about 8 minutes.

3. Add grated tomato and continue to cook for further 2 - 3 minutes.

4. Pour the broth and water. Bring to a boil, lower heat to low, cover and simmer for 20 minutes or until cabbage softened.

5. Sprinkle with ground black pepper, stir and serve.

Nutrition:

- Calories 155

- Total Fats 2g

- Carbs: 28g

- Protein 4g

- Dietary Fiber: 2.3g

Spinach Soup with Shiitake mushrooms

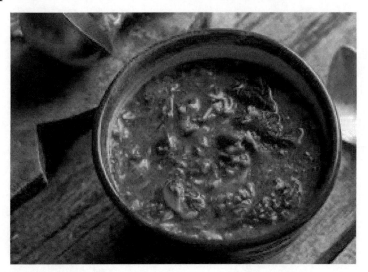

Preparation Time: 10 minutes

Cooking Time:15 minutes

Servings: 6

Ingredients:

- Tablespoon of olive oil

- 1 medium onion, chopped

- 2 cloves garlic, minced

- 2 cups of water

- 1/2 bunch of spinach

- 2 cups shiitake mushrooms, chopped

- 2 Tablespoon of almond flour

- 1 Tablespoon of coconut aminos

- 1 teaspoon coriander dry

- 1/2 teaspoon of ground mustard

- Salt and ground black pepper to taste

Directions:

1. Heat the olive oil and sauté the garlic and onion until golden brown.

2. Add the coconut aminos and the mushrooms and stir for a few minutes.

3. Pour water, chopped spinach and all remaining ingredients.

4. Cover and cook for 5 - 6 minutes or until spinach is tender.

5. Taste and adjust salt and the pepper.

6. Stir for further 5 minutes and remove for the heat.

7. Serve hot.

Nutrition:

- Calories 214

- Total Fats 2g

- Carbs: 24g

- Protein 10g

- Dietary Fiber: 2.3g

Vegan Artichoke Soup

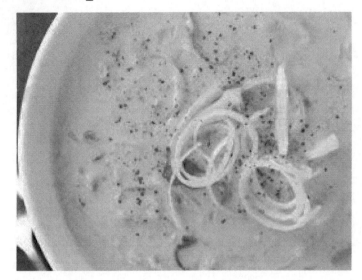

Preparation Time: 15 minutes

Cooking Time: 1 hour 5 minutes

Servings: 6

Ingredients:

- 1 Tablespoon of butter

- 2 artichoke hearts, halved

- 2 cloves garlic, minced

- 1 small onion, chopped

- 1 cup bone broth

- 2 cups of water

- 2 Tablespoon of almond flour

- Salt and ground black pepper to taste

- 2 Tablespoon of olive oil

- Fresh chopped parsley to taste

- Fresh chopped fresh basil to taste

Directions:

1. Heat the butter in a large pot, and add artichoke hearts, garlic and chopped onion.

2. Stir and cook until artichoke hearts tender.

3. Add bone broth, water and almond flout: season with the salt and pepper.

4. Bring soup to boil and cook for 2 minutes.

5. Add little olive oil, parsley and basil, stir and cook uncovered for 1 hour.

6. When ready, push the soup through sieve.

7. Taste and adjust salt and pepper.

8. Serve.

Nutrition:

- Calories: 252
- Carbohydrates: 21.9g
- Protein: 4.5g
- Fat: 17.7g
- Sugar: 0g
- Sodium: 58mg

Seafood Soup

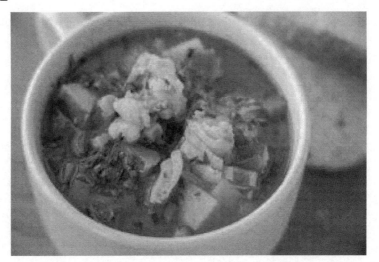

Preparation Time: 10 minutes

Cooking Time:25 minutes

Servings: 6

Ingredients:

- 1/2 cup of olive oil

- 1 spring onion cut in cubes

- Tablespoon of fresh celery, chopped

- 2 cloves of garlic minced

- 1 tomato, peeled and grated

- 2 bay leaves

- 1 teaspoon of anise

- 6 Large, raw shrimps

- 1 sea bass and 1 sea bream fillets cut in pieces; about 1 1/2 lbs.

- 1 lb. mussels, rinsed in plenty of cold water

- Salt and ground black pepper

- Tablespoon of chopped parsley for serving

- 6 cups of water

Directions:

1. Heat the olive oil in a large pot and sauté in the onion, garlic and celery for 4 -5 minutes over medium heat.

2. Add bay leaves, anise and grated tomato; stir and cook for further 5 minutes.

3. Add seafood and fish and pour 6 cups of water; season with little salt and pepper.

4. Cover and cook for 10 - 12 minutes on low heat. Serve hot with chopped parsley.

Nutrition:

- Calories: 546

- Carbohydrates: 21.9g

- Protein: 18.6g

- Fat: 43.1g

- Sugar: 0.8g

- Sodium: 678mg

Hot Spicy Chicken

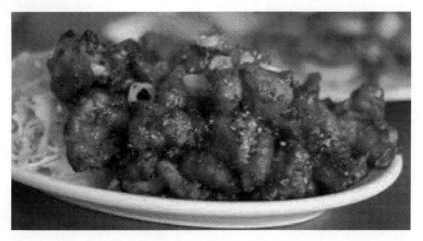

Preparation time: 5 minutes
Cooking time: 25 minutes

Servings: 6

Ingredients

- ¼ tbsp fennel seeds, ground

- ¼ tsp smoked paprika

- ½ tsp hot paprika

- ½ tsp minced garlic

- 2 chicken thighs, boneless

Directions

1. Turn on the oven, then set it to 325 degrees F and let it preheat.

2. Prepare the spice mix and for this, bring out a small bowl, add all the ingredients in it, except for chicken, and stir until well mixed.

3. Brush the mixture on all sides of the chicken, rub it well into the meat, then place chicken onto a baking sheet and roast for 15 to 25 minutes until thoroughly cooked, basting every 10 minutes with the drippings.

Nutrition: Calories: 205 - Carbohydrates: 36.2g - Protein: 4.3g - Fat: 5.3g - Sugar: 2.8g - Sodium: 463mg

Broccoli and Turkey Dish

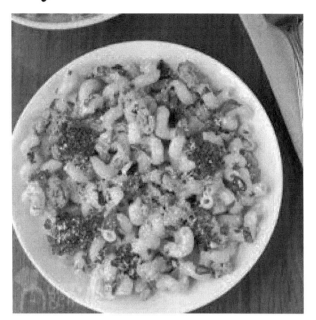

Preparation time: 5 minutes
Cooking time: 15 minutes

Servings: 6

Ingredients

- ¼ tsp red pepper flakes

- 1 tbsp olive oil

- 1 tsp soy sauce

- 4 oz broccoli florets

- 4 oz cauliflower florets, riced

- 4 oz ground turkey

Directions

1. Bring out a skillet pan, place it over medium heat, add olive oil and when hot, add beef, crumble it and cook for 8 minutes until no longer pink.

2. Then add broccoli florets and riced cauliflower, stir well, drizzle with soy sauce and sesame oil, season with salt, black pepper, and red pepper flakes and continue cooking for 5 minutes until vegetables have thoroughly cooked.

Nutrition:

- Calories – 263
- Fat – 14g
- Saturated Fat – 2g
- Trans Fat – 0g
- Carbohydrates – 36g
- Fiber – 11g
- Sodium – 168mg
- Protein – 5g

Easy Mayo Salmon

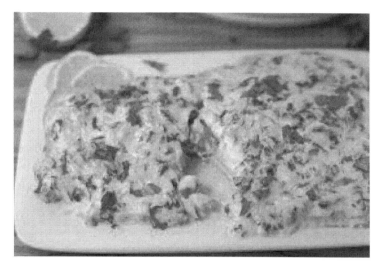

Preparation time: 5 minutes
Cooking time: 10 minutes

Servings: 6

Ingredients

- 2 salmon fillets

- 4 tbsp mayonnaise

Directions

1. Turn on the Panini press, spray it with oil and let it preheat.

2. Then spread 1 tbsp of mayonnaise on each side of salmon, place them on Panini press pan, shut with lid, and cook for 7 to 10 minutes until salmon has cooked to the desired level.

Nutrition

- Calories - 203

- Fat – 7g

- Carbohydrates – 33g

- Fiber – 2g

- Protein – 4.5g

Zesty Avocado and Lettuce Salad

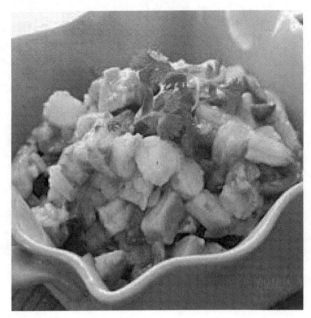

Preparation time: 5 minutes
Cooking time: 0 minutes

Servings: 6

Ingredients

- ½ of a lime, juiced

- 1 avocado, pitted, sliced

- 2 tbsp olive oil

- 4 oz chopped lettuce

- 4 tbsp chopped chives

Directions

1. Prepare the dressing and for this, bring out a small bowl, add oil, lime juice, salt, and black pepper, stir until mixed, and then slowly mix oil until combined.

2. Bring out a large bowl, add avocado, lettuce, and chives, and then toss gently.

3. Drizzle with dressing, toss until well coated, and then serve.

Nutrition: Calories 170 - Fat: 13.8g - Carbo: 3.4g - Dietary Fiber: 1.4g - Protein: 9.7g

Veggie, Bacon and Egg Dish

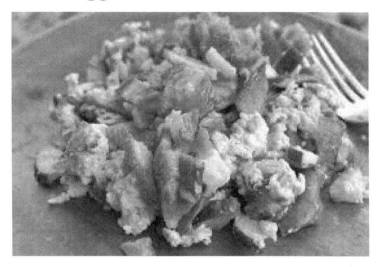

Preparation time: 5 minutes
Cooking time: 5 minutes

Servings: 6

Ingredients

- ¼ cup mayonnaise

- 2 eggs, boiled, sliced

- 4 oz spinach

- 4 slices of bacon, chopped

Directions

1. Bring out a skillet pan, place it over medium heat, add bacon, and cook for 5 minutes until browned.

2. In the meantime, bring out a salad bowl, add spinach in it, top with bacon and eggs and drizzle with mayonnaise.

3. Toss until well mixed and then serve.

Nutrition: Calories 63 - Fat: 4.4g - Carbohydrates: 0.3g - Dietary Fiber: 0g - Protein: 5.5g

Keto Teriyaki Chicken

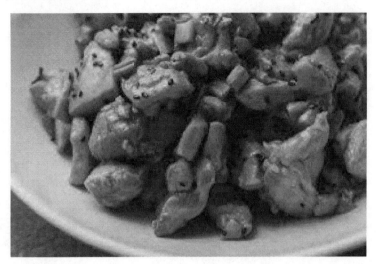

Preparation time: 5 minutes
Cooking time: 18 minutes

Servings: 6

Ingredients

- 1 tbsp olive oil
- 1 tbsp swerve sweetener
- 2 chicken thighs, boneless
- 2 tbsp soy sauce

Directions

1. Bring out a skillet pan, place it over medium heat, add oil and when hot, add chicken thighs and cook for 5 minutes per side until seared.

2. Then sprinkle sugar over chicken thighs, drizzle with soy sauce and bring the sauce to boil.

3. Switch heat to medium-low level, continue cooking for 3 minutes until chicken is evenly glazed, and then transfer to a plate.

4. Serve chicken with cauliflower rice.

Nutrition: Calories 471 - Fat: 31.7g - Carbo: 4.3g - Dietary Fiber: 1.3g - Protein: 42.9g

Low Carb Keto Pasta and Tomato sauce

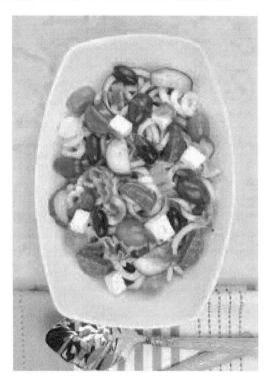

Preparation time: 40 minutes
Cooking time: 7 minutes

Servings: 6

Ingredients

- ¼ tsp ground black pepper

- ¼ tsp salt

- 2 egg yolks

- 2 tbsp tomato sauce

- 4 oz grated mozzarella cheese

Directions

1. Bring out a heatproof bowl, add mozzarella in it, and microwave for 2 minutes or until it melts.

2. Whisk in yolks until combined, bring out a baking dish lined with parchment paper, and add cheese mixture in it.

3. Cover the cheese mixture with another parchment paper, press and spread the cheese mixture as thinly as possible, let it rest for 10 minutes until slightly firm.

4. Then uncover it, cut out thin spaghetti by using a knife and refrigerate the pasta for 45 minutes.

5. When ready to cook, bring out a saucepan half full of salty water, bring it to boil, add pasta and cook for 5 minutes until spaghetti is tender.

6. Drain the spaghetti, distribute it between two bowls, top with tomato sauce, season with salt and black pepper, toss until well mixed, and then serve.

Nutrition:

- Calories 641
- Fat: 15g
- Carbohydrates 16.4g
- Fiber 6g
- Protein 14.43g

Lemon Garlic Shrimp Pasta

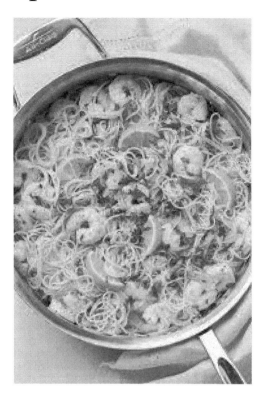

Preparation Time: 10 minutes

Cooking Time: 15 minutes

Servings: 4

Ingredients:

- Linguine pasta (2 bags)

- Garlic cloves (4)

- Olive oil (2 tbsp.)

- Butter (2 tbsp.)

- Lemon (.5 of 1)

- Large raw shrimp (1 lb.)

- Paprika (.5 tsp.)

- Fresh basil (as desired)

- Pepper and salt (as desired)

Directions:

1. Drain the water from the package of noodles and rinse them in cold water. Add them to a pot of boiling water for two minutes. Transfer to a hot skillet over medium heat to remove the excess liquid (dry roast). Set them aside.

2. Use the same pan to warm the butter, oil, and mashed garlic. Sauté for a few minutes, but don't brown.

3. Slice the lemon into rounds and add them to the garlic along with the shrimp. Sauté for approximately three minutes per side.

4. Add the noodles and spices and stir to blend the flavors.

Nutrition:

- Calories 281.93

- Fat 29.14g

- Carbohydrates 6.76g

- Fiber 2.04

- Protein 2.83g

Easy Spicy Beans

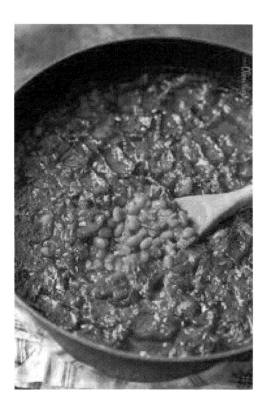

Preparation time: 5 minutes
Cooking time: 10 minutes

Servings: 6

Ingredients

- ¼ tsp crushed red pepper

- ½ tsp minced garlic

- 1 ½ tbsp olive oil

- 4 oz green beans

Directions

1. Bring out a saucepan half full of salted water, place it over medium heat, bring the water to boil, then add green beans and cook for 4 minutes until tender.

2. Drain the beans, wipe the pan, return it over medium heat, add oil and when hot, add garlic and cook for 1 minute until fragrant.

3. Then add green beans, season with salt and black pepper, cook for 1 minute and transfer beans to a plate.

4. Sprinkle red pepper on the green beans and serve.

Lime Chicken with Coleslaw

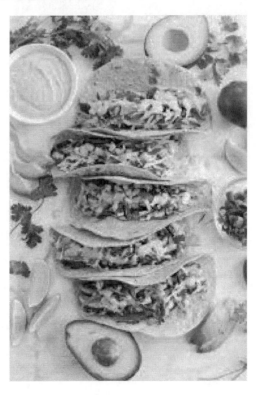

Preparation time: 35 minutes
Cooking time: 8 minutes

Servings: 6

Ingredients

- ¼ tsp minced garlic

- ½ of a lime, juiced, zested

- ¾ tbsp apple cider vinegar

- 1 chicken thigh, boneless

- 2 oz coleslaw

Directions

1. Prepare the marinade and for this, bring out a medium bowl, add vinegar, oil, garlic, paprika, salt, lime juice, and zest and stir until well mixed.

2. Cut chicken thighs into bite-size pieces, toss until well mixed, and marinate it in the refrigerator for 30 minutes.

3. Then Bring out a skillet pan, place it over medium-high heat, add butter and marinated chicken pieces and cook for 8 minutes until golden brown and thoroughly cooked.

4. Serve chicken with coleslaw.

Nutrition:

- Calories 400

- Total Fats 30g

- Carbs: 9g

- Protein 20g

- Dietary Fiber: 0.8g

Spinach and Tuna Salad

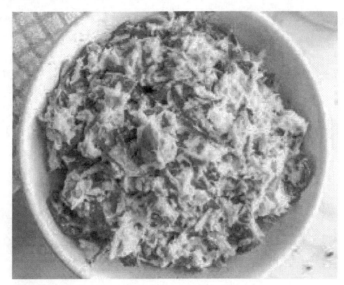

Preparation time: 5 minutes
Cooking time: 0 minutes

Servings: 6

Ingredients

- 1 tbsp grated mozzarella cheese

- 1/3 cup mayonnaise

- 2 oz chopped spinach

- 4 oz tuna, packed in water

Directions

1. Bring out a bowl, add mayonnaise in it along with cheese, season with salt and black pepper and whisk until combined.

2. Then add tuna and spinach, toss until mixed and serve.

Nutrition:

- Calories 337

- Fat 18.1 g

- Carbohydrates 40.3 g

- Sugar 13.7 g

- Protein 6.4 g

- Cholesterol 0 mg

Sautéed Sausage and Beans

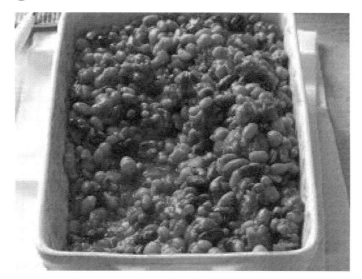

Preparation time: 5 minutes
Cooking time: 4 minutes

Servings: 6

Ingredients

- ¼ tsp dried oregano

- 1 cup of water

- 1 tbsp olive oil

- 4 oz chicken sausage, sliced

- 4 oz green beans

Directions

1. Turn on the instant pot, place all the ingredients in the inner pot, stir and shut with lid.

2. Press the manual button, cook for 4 minutes at high-pressure setting, and, when done, do quick pressure release.

Grilled Chicken with Spinach and Mozzarella

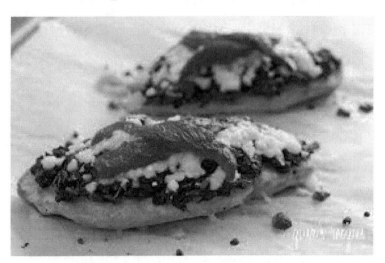

Preparation Time: 20 minutes

Cooking Time: 40 minutes

Servings: 6

Ingredients:

- Large chicken breasts (24 oz. or 6 portions)

- Olive oil (1 tsp.)

- Pepper and Kosher salt (as desired)

- Garlic cloves (3 crushed)

- Drained frozen spinach (10 oz.)

- Roasted red pepper strips packed in water (.5 cup)

- Shredded part-skim mozzarella (3 oz.)

- Olive oil cooking spray

Directions:

1. Warm the oven to 400° Fahrenheit.

2. Prepare the grill/grill pan with the oil.

3. Sprinkle the salt and pepper onto the chicken. Cook about two to three minutes per side.

4. Add the oil into a frying pan along with the garlic. Continue cooking for about 30 seconds, add a sprinkle of salt and pepper, and toss in the spinach. Sauté another two to three minutes.

5. Arrange the chicken on a baking sheet and add the spinach to each one. Top them off with half of the cheese and peppers. Bake for about three minutes until lightly toasted.

6. Serve.

Nutrition:

- Calories 392

- Fat 29 g

- Carbohydrates 32.6 g

- Sugar 13.7 g

- Protein 4.6 g

- Cholesterol 1 mg

Cheese and Bacon Stuffed Zucchini

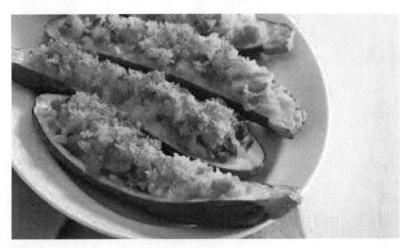

Preparation time: 5 minutes
Cooking time: 20 minutes

Servings: 6

Ingredients

- 1 tbsp chopped spinach

- 1 tbsp grated mozzarella cheese

- 1 zucchini, halved lengthwise

- 2 slices of bacon

- 3 tbsp cream cheese

Directions

1. Turn on the oven, then set it to 350 degrees F and let it preheat.

2. In the meantime, cut zucchini into half lengthwise, then use a spoon to remove the seedy center and set aside until required.

3. Place remaining ingredients, except for bacon in a bowl, stir well, and then evenly stuffed this mixture into zucchini.

4. Wrap each zucchini half with a bacon slice, place them on a baking sheet lined with parchment paper and cook for 15 to 20 minutes until zucchini is tender and bacon is browned.

Nutrition:

- Calories 255

- Fat 5 g

- Carbohydrates 44.9 g

- Sugar 17.1 g

- Protein 9.2 g

- Cholesterol 9 mg

Chicken and Greens Soup

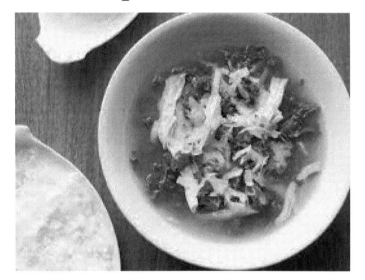

Preparation Time: 12 minutes

Cooking Time:1 hour 50 minutes

Servings: 8

Ingredients:

- 1/4 cup of olive oil

- 1 1/2 lbs. chicken breast, boneless, cut into cube

- 1 spring onion, cut into cubes

- 1 clove of garlic, finely chopped

- 1 1/2 lettuce cos or romain, chopped

- 1 cup of fresh spinach finely chopped

- 1 bunch of dill finely chopped, without the thick stalks

- 1/2 Tablespoon of sweet chill powder

- 1 teaspoon of fresh mint, chopped

- 1 teaspoon of fresh thyme, chopped

- Salt and freshly ground pepper

- 5 cups of water

Directions:

1. In a deep pot, heat the olive oil to a high heat and sauté the chicken for about 5 - 6 minutes.

2. Add the onion and sauté for about 3 minutes until softened.

3. Add the garlic, the lettuce, spinach, dill, mint, thyme and sauté for about 3-4 minutes, stirring with a wooden spoon.

4. Sprinkle with chili, salt, freshly ground pepper and pour 5 cups of water.

5. Bring to boil and cook for 1 1/2 hours on low heat.

6. Serve hot.

Nutrition:

- Calories: 122

- Carbohydrates: 11.5g

- Protein: 5.1g

- Fat: 8g

- Sugar: 2.8g

- Sodium: 69mg

Cold Cauliflower and Cilantro Soup

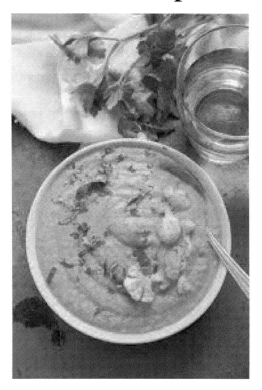

Preparation Time: 5 minutes

Cooking Time:25 minutes

Servings: 8

Ingredients:

- 1 1/2 lbs. cauliflower previously steamed

- 1 cup almond milk

- 1/2 teaspoon fresh ginger grated

- 2 bunches fresh cilantro

- Tablespoon garlic-infused olive oil

- pinch of salt

Directions:

1. Heat water in a large pot until boiling. Place the steamer in a pot and put in the cauliflower.

2. Cover and steam cauliflower for 6 - 7 minutes.

3. Remove the cauliflower along with all ingredients from the list above in a high-speed blender.

4. Blend until smooth or until desired texture is achieved.

5. Pour the soup in a glass container, cover and refrigerate for 2 - 3 hours.

6. Serve cold.

Nutrition:

- Calories: 293

- Carbohydrates: 24.7g

- Protein: 3.8g

- Fat: 21.2g

- Sugar: 2.9g

- Sodium: 223mg

Creamy Broccoli Soup with Nutmeg

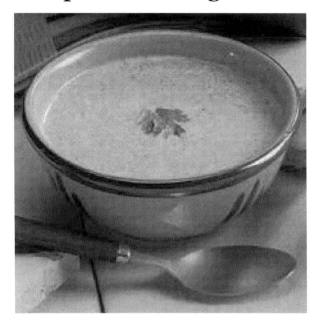

Preparation Time: 15 minutes

Cooking Time: 20 minutes

Servings: 8

Ingredients:

- Tablespoon of olive oil

- 2 green onions finely chopped

- 1 lb. broccoli floret, frozen or fresh

- 1 cups of bone broth cold

- 1 cup of cream

- Salt and ground pepper to taste

- 1 Tablespoon of nutmeg

Directions:

1. Heat the olive oil in a pot over medium-high heat.

2. Add the onion in and sauté it until becomes translucent.

3. Add the broccoli, season with the salt and pepper, and bring to boil.

4. Cover the pot and cook for 6 - 8 minutes.

5. Transfer the broccoli mixture into blender, and blend until smooth.

6. Pour the cream, and blend for further 30 seconds.

7. Return the soup in a pot and reheat it.

8. Adjust salt and pepper and serve hot with grated nutmeg.

Nutrition:

- Calories 165
- Fat 2.8 g
- Carbohydrates 30.9 g
- Sugar 13.6 g
- Protein 5.3 g
- Cholesterol 5 mg

Creamy Mushroom Soup with Crumbled Bacon

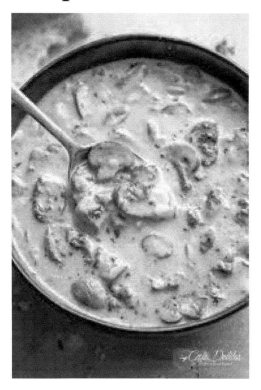

Preparation Time: 15 minutes

Cooking Time:55 minutes

Servings: 8

Ingredients:

- 1 Tablespoon of lard

- 1 and ½ lbs. of white mushrooms

- 1/2 cup of water

- 1/2 cups of almond milk

- 2 green onions, finely sliced

- 3 sprigs of fresh rosemary

- 2 cloves garlic, finely chopped

- slices of bacon, fried and crumbled

- Salt and ground black pepper

Directions:

1. Heat the lard in a large skillet and sauté green onions and garlic over medium-high heat.

2. Season with the salt and pepper, and rosemary; pour water and cook for 5 minutes.

3. Add the mushrooms and sauté for 1-2 minutes.

4. Pour the almond milk, stir, cover and simmer for 40 minutes over low heat.

5. Remove the rosemary and transfer the soup in your blender; blend until creamy and soft.

6. Adjust salt, and if necessary, add some warm water.

7. Chop the bacon and fry in a hot pan until it becomes crisp.

8. Serve your soup in bowls and sprinkle with chopped bacon.

Nutrition:

- Calories 130

- Fat 3.9 g

- Carbohydrates 21.2 g

- Sugar 10.4 g

- Protein 3.9 g

- Cholesterol 6 mg

Creamy Mushroom and Zucchini Soup

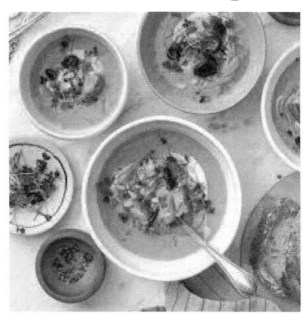

Preparation and Cooking time: 40 minutes

Servings: 8

Ingredients:

- 1 large zucchini, chopped

- 1 lb. fresh mushrooms, chopped

- 3 cups chicken or vegetable stock

- 1 medium onion, chopped

- 2 cloves garlic, minced

- 2 bay leaves

- 1 tablespoon dried thyme

- 1 tablespoon ghee

- 1 cup coconut milk

- Sea salt

- Freshly ground black pepper

Directions:

1. Place a large saucepan over medium heat and melt the ghee. Add the onions and garlic. Sauté about 3 minutes.

2. Add the mushrooms, bay leaves, and thyme. Cook an additional 4 minutes.

3. Add the zucchini and cook until the vegetables release their juices.

4. Add the stock to the pan and bring it to a boil. Reduce the heat and let it simmer about 5 minutes.

5. Discard the bay leaves and add the coconut milk. Simmer another 5 minutes, stirring the mixture frequently.

6. Transfer the soup to a blender in batches and process until smooth. If you have an immersion blender, you can use it. Serve warm.

Nutrition:

- Calories 195
- Fat 11.2 g
- Carbohydrates 20.1 g
- Sugar 4.3 g
- Protein 5.5 g
- Cholesterol 0 mg

Creamy Cauliflower Chowder

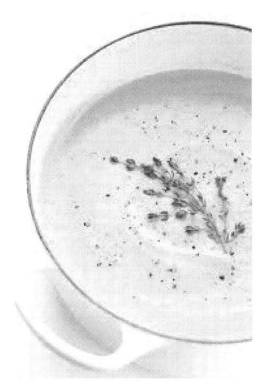

Preparation and Cooking Time: 20-25 minutes

Servings: 8

Ingredients:

- 1 head of cauliflower cut into small florets
- ¾ cup diced carrots
- ½ cup diced onion
- 1 cup milk
- 1 tablespoon butter
- ¼ cup cream cheese
- 5 cloves of garlic, minced
- ½ teaspoon dried oregano
- 1 teaspoon freshly ground pepper

- salt to taste

- 1 cup of water

- 1 tablespoon of olive oil and 3 oz of shredded cheddar cheese for topping

Directions:

1. Heat butter in a soup pot.

2. Add onion and garlic and sauté for a few minutes.

3. Add cauliflower, carrots, milk, pepper, salt, and oregano.

4. Bring this mixture to boil and then reduce heat to a simmer.

5. After the cauliflower is tender, remove soup pot from heat and pour the mixture into a blender.

6. Blend soup until creamy then pour it back in the pot.

7. Add a cup of water along with cream cheese.

8. Simmer for 5 to 10 minutes and then turn off heat.

9. Top with olive oil and shredded cheddar.

Nutrition:

- Calories 208

- Fat 10.4 g

- Carbohydrates 6.3 g

- Sugar 4.1 g

- Protein 21.7 g

- Cholesterol 33 mg

DINNER

Chicken Meatloaf Cups with Pancetta

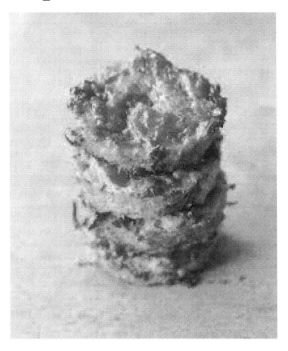

Preparation Time: 10 minutes

Cooking Time: 25 minutes

Servings: 6

Ingredients

- 2 tbsp onion, chopped

- 1 tsp garlic, minced

- 1 pound ground chicken

- 2 ounces cooked pancetta, chopped

- 1 egg, beaten

- 1 tsp mustard

- Salt and black pepper, to taste

- ½ tsp crushed red pepper flakes

- 1 tsp dried basil

- ½ tsp dried oregano

- 4 ounces cheddar cheese, cubed

Directions

1. In a bowl, mix mustard, onion, ground chicken, egg, pancetta, and garlic. Season with oregano, red pepper, black pepper, basil and salt.

2. Split the mixture into greased muffin cups. Lower one cube of cheddar cheese into each meatloaf cup.

3. Close the top to cover the cheese. Bake in the oven at 345°F for 20 minutes, or until the meatloaf cups become golden brown.

4. Let cool for 10 minutes before transferring from the muffin pan.

Nutrition:

- Calories 237

- Fat 4.5 g

- Carbohydrates 37.5 g

- Sugar 1.9 g

- Protein 13.2 g

- Cholesterol 0 mg

Ham and Emmental Eggs

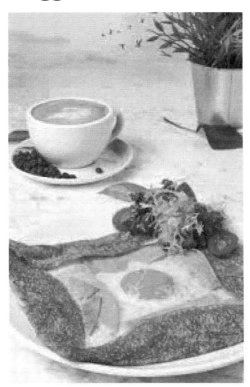

Preparation Time: 10 minutes

Cooking Time:35 minutes

Servings: 6

Ingredients

- 1 tbsp olive oil

- 4 slices ham, chopped

- ½ cup chives, chopped

- ½ cup broccoli, chopped

- 1 clove garlic, minced

- 1 tsp fines herbs

- ¼ cup vegetable broth

- 5 eggs

- 1 ½ cups Emmental cheese, shredded

Directions

1. In a frying pan, warm oil. Add in ham and cook for 4 minutes, until brown and crispy; set aside.

2. Using the same pan, cook chives. Place in the garlic and broccoli and cook until soft as you stir occasionally. Stir in broth and fines herbs and cook for 6 more minutes.

3. Make 5 holes in the mixture until you are able to see the bottom of your pan.

4. Crack an egg into each hole. Spread cheese over the top and cook for 6 more minutes. Scatter the reserved ham over to serve.

Nutrition:

- Calories 450

- Fat 4.3 g

- Carbohydrates 72.6 g

- Sugar 2.6 g

- Protein 29.9 g

- Cholesterol 19 mg

Chorizo and Cheese Gofre

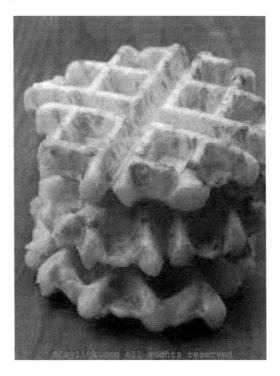

Preparation Time: 10 minutes

Cooking Time: 20 minutes

Servings: 6

Ingredients

- 6 eggs, separate egg whites and egg yolks

- ½ tsp baking powder

- 6 tbsp almond flour

- 4 tbsp butter, melted

- ¼ tsp salt

- ½ tsp dried rosemary

- 3 tbsp tomato puree

- 3 ounces smoked chorizo, chopped

- 3 ounces cheddar cheese, shredded

Directions

1. In a mixing bowl, mix egg yolks, almond flour, rosemary, butter, baking powder, and salt. Beat the egg whites until pale and combine with the egg yolk mixture.

2. Grease waffle iron and set over medium heat, add in ¼ cup of the batter and cook for 3 minutes until golden. Repeat with the remaining batter.

3. Place one waffle back to the waffle iron; sprinkle 1 tbsp of tomato puree to the waffle; apply a topping of 1 ounce of cheese and 1 ounce of chorizo. Cover with another waffle Cooking until all the cheese melts.

4. Do the same with all remaining ingredients.

Nutrition:

- Calories 244
- Fat 5.7 g
- Carbohydrates 37.1 g
- Sugar 13.2 g
- Protein 11.4 g
- Cholesterol 10 mg

Cheese, Ham and Egg Muffins

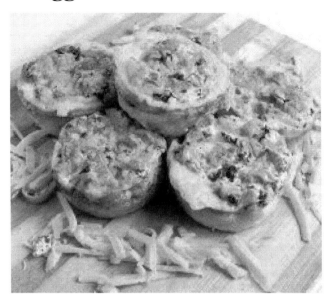

Preparation Time: 10 minutes

Cooking Time:30 minutes

Servings: 6

Ingredients

- 24 slices smoked ham

- 6 eggs, beaten

- Salt and black pepper, to taste

- ¼ cup fresh parsley, chopped

- ¼ cup ricotta cheese

- ¼ cup Brie, chopped

Directions

1. Set oven to 390°F. Line 2 slices of smoked ham into each greased muffin cup, to circle each mold. In a mixing bowl, mix the rest of the ingredients.

2. Fill ¾ of the ham lined muffin cup with the egg/cheese mixture. Bake for 15 minutes. Serve warm!

Nutrition: Kcal 279 - Carbs 28g - Fat 6g - Protein 17g

Baked Chicken Legs with Cheesy Spread

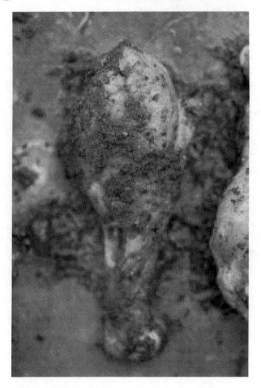

Preparation Time: 10 minutes

Cooking Time: 20 minutes

Servings: 6

Ingredients

- 4 chicken legs

- ¼ cup goat cheese

- 2 tbsp sour cream

- 1 tbsp butter, softened

- 1 onion, chopped

- Sea salt and black pepper, to taste

Directions

1. Preheat oven to 360°F and season the legs with salt and black pepper.

2. Roast in a greased baking dish for 25-30 minutes until crispy and browned.

3. In a mixing bowl, mix the rest of the ingredients to form the spread. Scatter the spread over the chicken and serve with green salad.

Nutrition:

- Kcal 510

- Carbs 54g

- Fat 21g

- Protein 36g

Quattro Formaggio Pizza

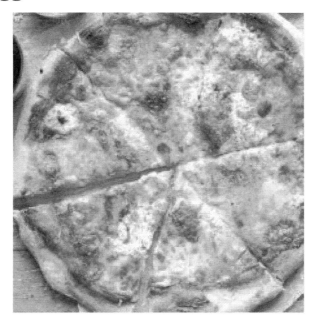

Preparation Time: 10 minutes

Cooking Time: 40 minutes

Servings: 6

Ingredients

- 1 tbsp olive oil

- ½ cup cheddar cheese, shredded

- 1 ¼ cups mozzarella cheese, shredded

- ½ cup mascarpone cheese

- ½ cup blue cheese

- 2 tbsp sour cream

- 2 garlic cloves, chopped

- 1 red bell pepper, sliced

- 1 green bell pepper, sliced

- 10 cherry tomatoes, halved

- 1 tsp oregano

- Salt and black pepper, to taste

Directions

1. In a bowl, mix the cheeses. Set a pan over medium heat and warm olive oil.

2. Spread the cheese mixture on the pan and cook for 5 minutes until cooked through. Scatter garlic and sour cream over the crust.

3. Add in tomatoes and bell peppers Cooking for 2 minutes. Sprinkle with pepper, salt and oregano and serve.

Herbal Green Beans and Chicken

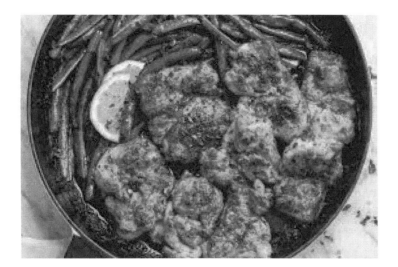

Preparation Time: 15 minutes

Cooking Time: 35 minutes

Servings: 3

Ingredients:

- Olive oil (2 tbsp.)

- Trimmed green beans (1 cup)

- Whole chicken breasts (2)

- Cherry tomatoes (8 halve)

- Italian seasoning (1 tbsp.)

- Salt and pepper (1 tsp. of each)

Directions:

1. Warm a skillet using the medium heat setting; add the oil.

2. Sprinkle the chicken with the pepper, Italian seasoning, and salt.

3. Arrange in the skillet for 10 minutes per side – or until thoroughly done.

4. Add the tomatoes and beans. Simmer another 5 to 7 minutes and serve.

Nutrition: Kcal 336 - Carbs 43g - Fat 13g - Protein 15g

Bacon Balls with Brie Cheese

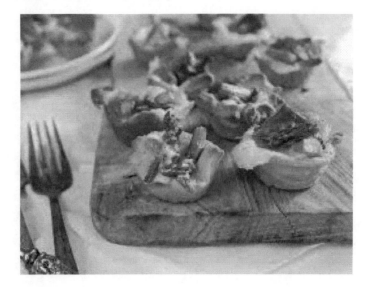

Preparation Time: 10 minutes

Cooking Time: 40 minutes

Servings: 6

Ingredients

- 3 ounces bacon
- 6 ounces brie cheese
- 1 chili pepper, seeded and chopped
- ¼ tsp parsley flakes
- ½ tsp paprika

Directions

1. Set a pan over medium heat and fry the bacon until crispy; then crush it.

2. Place the other ingredients in a bowl and mix to combine with the bacon grease. Refrigerate the mixture for 20 minutes. Remove and form balls from the mixture.

3. Set the bacon in a plate and roll the balls around to coat.

Nutrition: Calories 456 - Total Fats 18g - Carbs: 41g - Protein 17g - Dietary Fiber: 1.8g

Creamy Cheddar Deviled Eggs

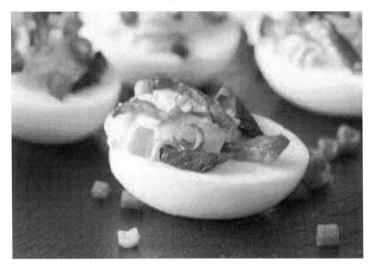

Preparation Time: 10 minutes

Cooking Time: 20 minutes

Servings: 6

Ingredients

- 10 eggs

- ¼ cup mayonnaise

- 1 tbsp tomato paste

- 2 tbsp celery, chopped

- 2 tbsp carrot, chopped

- 2 tbsp chives, minced

- 2 tbsp cheddar cheese, grated

- Salt and black pepper, to taste

Directions

1. Place the eggs in a pot and fill with water by about 1 inch. Bring the eggs to a boil over high heat, then reduce the heat to medium and simmer for 10 minutes.

2. Remove and rinse under running water until cooled. Peel and discard the shell. Slice each egg in half lengthwise and get rid of the yolks.

3. Mix the yolks with the rest of the ingredients. Split the mixture amongst the egg whites and set deviled eggs on a plate to serve.

Nutrition:

- Calories 156

- Fat 2.6 g

- Carbohydrates 1.5 g

- Sugar 0.1 g

- Protein 29 g

- Cholesterol 213 mg

Jamon & Queso Balls

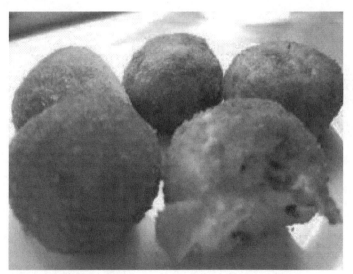

Preparation Time: 10 minutes

Cooking Time:30 minutes

Servings: 6

Ingredients

- 1 egg

- 6 slices jamon serrano, chopped

- 6 ounces cotija cheese

- 6 ounces Manchego cheese

- Salt and black pepper, to taste

- ¼ cup almond flour

- 1 tsp baking powder

- 1 tsp garlic powder

Directions

1. Preheat oven to 420 °F.

2. Whisk the egg; place in the remaining ingredients and mix well. Split the mixture into 16 balls;

3. Set the balls on a baking sheet lined with parchment paper.

4. Bake for 13 minutes or until they turn golden brown and become crispy.

Nutrition:

- Calories 185

- Total Fats 8.5g

- Carbs: 0g

- Protein 27g

- Dietary Fiber: 0g

Cajun Crabmeat Frittata

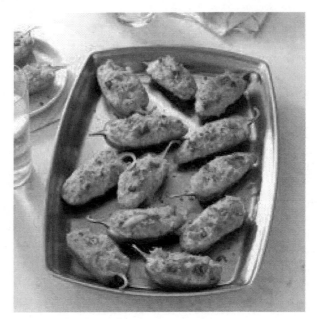

Preparation Time: 10 minutes

Cooking Time: 20 minutes

Servings: 6

Ingredients

- 1 tbsp olive oil

- 1 onion, chopped

- 4 ounces crabmeat, chopped

- 1 tsp cajun seasoning

- 6 large eggs, slightly beaten

- ½ cup Greek yogurt

Directions

1. Preheat oven to 350°F. Set a large skillet over medium heat and warm the oil. Add in onion and sauté until soft, about 3 minutes.

2. Stir in crabmeat and cook for 2 more minutes. Season with Cajun seasoning. Evenly distribute the ingredients at the bottom of the skillet.

3. Whisk the eggs with yogurt. Transfer to the skillet. Set the skillet in the oven and bake for about 18 minutes or until eggs are cooked through. Slice into wedges and serve warm.

Nutrition:

- Calories 280
- Total Fats 17g
- Carbs: 3g
- Protein 35g
- Dietary Fiber: 1g

Crabmeat & Cheese Stuffed Avocado

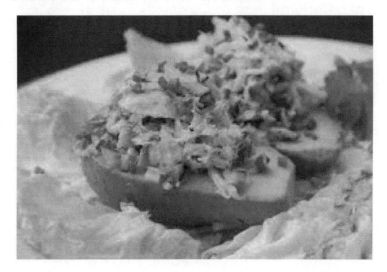

Preparation Time: 10 minutes

Cooking Time: 50 minutes

Servings: 6

Ingredients

- 1 tsp olive oil

- 1 cup crabmeat

- 2 avocados, halved and pitted

- 3 ounces cream cheese

- ¼ cup almonds, chopped

- 1 tsp smoked paprika

Directions

1. Preheat oven to 425ºF and grease a baking pan with cooking spray.

2. In a bowl, mix crabmeat with cream cheese. To the avocado halves, place in almonds and crabmeat/cheese mixture and bake for 18 minutes.

3. Decorate with smoked paprika and serve.

Nutrition: Calories 300 - Total Fats 8g - Carbs: 5g - Protein 18g - Dietary Fiber: 2g

Juicy Beef Cheeseburgers

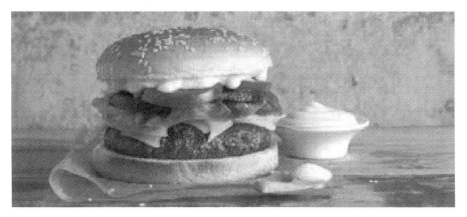

Preparation Time: 10 minutes

Cooking Time:20 minutes

Servings: 6

Ingredients

- 1 pound ground beef
- ½ cup green onions, chopped
- 2 garlic cloves, finely chopped
- ¼ tsp black pepper
- Salt and cayenne pepper, to taste
- 2 oz mascarpone cheese
- 3 oz pecorino Romano cheese, grated
- 2 tbsp olive oil

Directions

1. In a mixing bowl, mix ground beef, garlic, cayenne pepper, black pepper, green onions, and salt. Shape into 6 balls; then flatten to make burgers.

2. In a separate bowl, mix mascarpone with grated pecorino Romano cheeses. Split the cheese mixture among prepared patties.

3. Wrap the meat mixture around the cheese mixture to ensure that the filling is sealed inside. Warm oil in a skillet over medium heat.

4. Cook the burgers for 5 minutes each side.

Nutrition:

- Calories 130

- Total Fats 8g

- Carbs: 5g

- Protein 16g

- Dietary Fiber: 2g

Cilantro & Chili Omelet

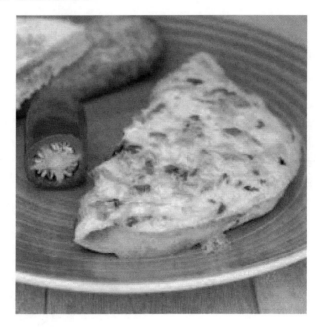

Preparation Time: 10 minutes

Cooking Time: 20 minutes

Servings: 6

Ingredients

- 2 tsp butter

- 2 spring onions, chopped

- 2 spring garlic, chopped

- 4 eggs

- 1 cup sour cream, divided

- 2 tomatoes, sliced

- 1 green chili pepper, minced

- 2 tbsp fresh cilantro, chopped

- Salt and black pepper, to taste

Directions

1. Set a pan over high heat and warm the butter. Sauté garlic and onions until tender and translucent.

2. Whisk the eggs with sour cream. Pour into the pan and use a spatula to smooth the surface

3. Cooking until eggs become puffy and brown to bottom. Add cilantro, chili pepper and tomatoes to one side of the omelet.

4. Season with black pepper and salt. Fold the omelet in half and slice into wedges.

Nutrition:

- Calories – 216

- Fat – 4g

- Saturated Fat – 1g

- Trans Fat – 0g

- Carbohydrates – 2g

- Fiber – 0g

- Sodium – 346mg

- Protein – 8g

Zucchini with Blue Cheese and Walnuts

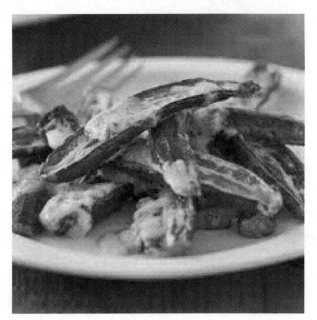

Preparation Time: 10 minutes

Cooking Time:60 minutes

Servings: 6

Ingredients

- 2 tbsp olive oil

- 6 zucchinis, sliced

- 1 ⅓ cups heavy cream

- 1 cup sour cream

- 8 ounces blue cheese

- 1 tsp Italian seasoning

- ¼ cup walnut halves

Directions

1. Set a grill pan over medium heat. Season zucchinis with Italian seasoning and drizzle with olive oil. Grill the zucchini until lightly charred. Remove to a serving platter.

2. In a dry pan over medium heat, toast the walnuts for 2-3 minutes and set aside.

3. Add the heavy cream, blue cheese, and sour cream to the pan and mix until everything is well combined.

4. Let cool for a few minutes and scatter over the grilled zucchini. Top with walnuts to serve.

Nutrition:

- Calories 181

- Total Fats 11.5g

- Carbs: 1.8g

- Protein 27.3g

- Dietary Fiber: 0.7g

Garlick & Cheese Turkey Slices

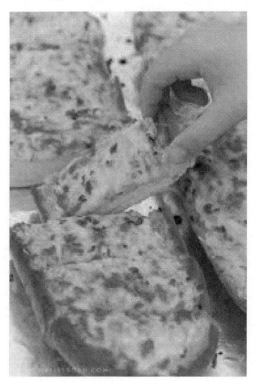

Preparation Time: 10 minutes

Cooking Time: 20 minutes

Servings: 6

Ingredients

- 2 tbsp olive oil

- 1 pound turkey breasts, sliced

- 2 garlic cloves, minced

- ½ cup heavy cream

- ⅓ cup chicken broth

- 2 tbsp tomato paste

- 1 cup cheddar cheese, shredded

Directions

1. Set a pan over medium heat and warm the oil; add in garlic and turkey and fry for 4 minutes; set aside.

2. Stir in the broth, tomato paste, and heavy cream Cooking until thickened.

3. Return the turkey to the pan; spread shredded cheddar cheese over.

4. Let sit for 5 minutes covered or until the cheese melts. Serve instantly

Nutrition:

- Calories 595
- Total Fats 31.5g
- Carbs: 52.6 g
- Protein 17.7g
- Dietary Fiber: 9.4g

Prosciutto & Cheese Egg Cups

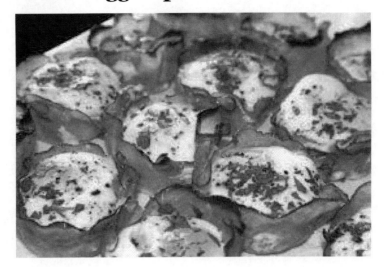

Preparation Time: 10 minutes

Cooking Time:60 minutes

Servings: 6

Ingredients

- 9 slices prosciutto

- 9 eggs

- 4 green onions, chopped

- ½ cup cheddar cheese, shredded

- ¼ tsp garlic powder

- ½ tsp dried dill weed

- Sea salt and black pepper, to taste

Directions

1. Preheat oven to 390°F and grease a 9-cup muffin pan with oil.

2. Line one slice of prosciutto on each cup. In a mixing bowl, combine the remaining ingredients.

3. Split the egg mixture among muffin cups. Bake for 20 minutes.

Nutrition:

- Calories 221

- Fat 9.1 g

- Carbohydrates 12 g

- Sugar 0.3 g

- Protein 21.9 g

- Cholesterol 174 mg

Spanish Salsa Aioli

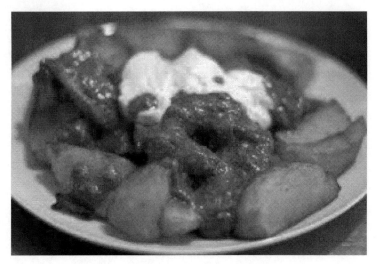

Preparation Time: 10 minutes

Cooking Time: 20 minutes

Servings: 6

Ingredients

- 1 tbsp lemon juice

- 1 egg yolk, at room temperature

- 1 clove garlic, crushed

- ½ tsp salt

- ½ cup olive oil

- ¼ tsp black pepper

- ¼ cup fresh parsley, chopped

Directions

1. Using a blender, place in salt, lemon juice, garlic, and egg yolk; pulse well to get a smooth and creamy mixture.

2. Set blender to slow speed.

3. Slowly sprinkle in olive oil and combine to ensure the oil incorporates well. Stir in parsley and black pepper.

4. Refrigerate the mixture until ready.

Nutrition:

- Calories 571

- Fat 35.1 g

- Carbohydrates 26 g

- Sugar 3.9 g

- Protein 36.9 g

- Cholesterol 133 mg

Three-Cheese Fondue with Walnuts and Parsley

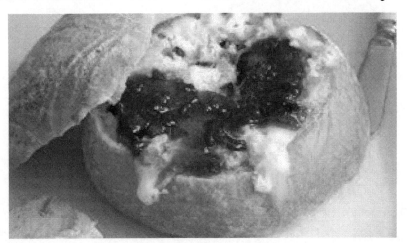

Preparation Time: 10 minutes

Cooking Time: 50 minutes

Servings: 6

Ingredients

- ½ pound brie cheese, chopped
- ⅓ pound Swiss cheese, shredded
- ½ cup Emmental cheese, grated
- 1 tbsp xanthan gum
- ½ tsp garlic powder
- 1 tsp onion powder
- ¾ cup white wine
- ½ tbsp lemon juice
- Black pepper, to taste
- 1 cup walnuts, chopped

Directions

1. Set broiler to preheat. In a skillet, thoroughly mix onion powder, brie, Emmental, Swiss cheese, garlic powder, and xanthan gum.

2. Pour in lemon juice and wine and sprinkle with black pepper.

3. Set the skillet under the broiler for 6 to 7 minutes, until the cheese browns. Garnish with walnuts.

Nutrition:

- Calories 290

- Fat 4.8 g

- Carbohydrates 40.1 g

- Sugar 5.2 g

- Protein 23.6 g

- Cholesterol 119 mg

Mushroom Salad

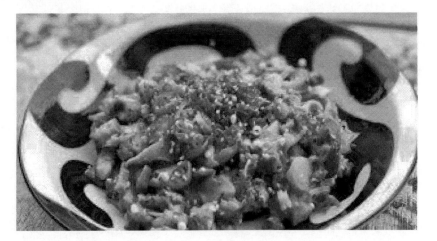

Preparation Time: 10 minutes

Cooking time: 10 minutes

Servings: 4

Ingredients:

- 2 tablespoons butter

- 1 pound cremini mushrooms, chopped

- 2 tablespoons extra virgin olive oil

- Salt and ground black pepper, to taste

- 2 bunches arugula

- 4 slices prosciutto

- 2 tablespoons apple cider vinegar

- sundried tomatoes in oil, drained, and chopped

- Parmesan cheese, shaved

- Fresh parsley leaves, chopped

Directions:

1. Heat a pan with butter and half of the oil over medium–high heat.

2. Add mushrooms, salt, and pepper, stir, and cook for 3 minutes. Reduce heat, stir again, and cook for 3 more minutes.

3. Add rest of the oil and vinegar, stir and cook 1 minute.

4. Place arugula on a serving platter, add prosciutto on top, add the mushroom mixture, sundried tomatoes, more salt and pepper, Parmesan shavings, parsley, and serve.

Nutrition:

- Calories 211

- Fat 9.7 g

- Carbohydrates 1.7 g

- Sugar 0 g

- Protein 29.7 g

- Cholesterol 67 mg

Greek Side Salad

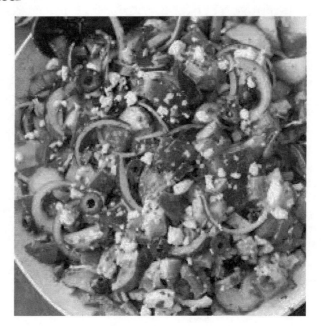

Preparation Time: 10 minutes

Cooking time: 7 minutes

Servings: 4

Ingredients:

- 1 and ½ pounds mushrooms, sliced

- 1 tablespoon extra-virgin olive oil

- 2 garlic cloves, peeled and minced

- 1 teaspoon dried basil

- Salt and ground black pepper, to taste

- 1 tomato, cored and diced

- 2 tablespoons lemon juice

- ½ cup water

- 1 tablespoons coriander, chopped

Directions:

1. Heat a pan with the oil over medium heat, add mushrooms, stir, and cook for 3 minutes.

2. Add basil and garlic, stir, and cook for 1 minute.

3. Add water, salt, pepper, tomato, and lemon juice, stir, and cook for a few minutes.

4. Take off heat, transfer to a bowl, set aside to cool down, sprinkle the coriander, and serve.

Nutrition:

- Calories 310
- Total Fats 13g
- Carbs: 10g
- Protein 40g
- Dietary Fiber: 3.5g

Tomato Salsa

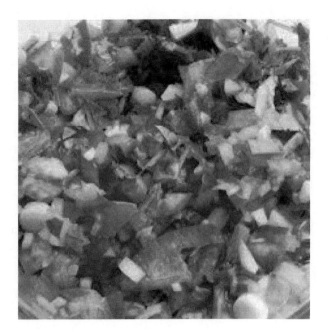

Preparation Time: 2 hours

Servings: 4

Ingredients:

- 3 yellow tomatoes, seeded and chopped
- 1 red tomato, seeded and chopped
- Salt and ground black pepper, to taste
- ⅓ cup onion, diced
- 1 jalapeño pepper, diced
- ¼ cup cilantro, diced
- 2 tablespoons lime juice
- 1/3 teaspoons stevia

Directions:

1. In a bowl, mix tomatoes with onion, and jalapeño.
2. Add cilantro, lime juice, salt, pepper, stevia, and stir well.
3. Cover the bowl, keep in the refrigerator for 2 hours, and serve.

Nutrition:

- Calories 150
- Total Fats 2g
- Carbs: 18g
- Protein 21g
- Dietary Fiber: 1g

Grilled Steak Salad

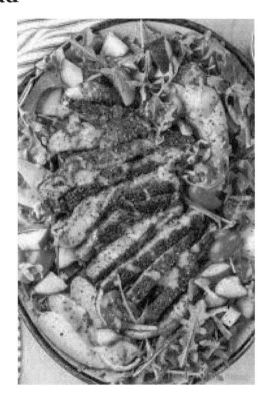

Preparation and Cooking time: 55 minutes

Servings: 4

Ingredients:

- 1 Cucumber, sliced
- 1 cup Halved cherry tomatoes
- 1 package Mixed greens

- 1 lb. Flank steak

- Soy sesame dressing

- 1 Grated carrot

Directions:

1. Take out a bowl and add in the steak with a drizzle of the dressing. Make sure that all your steak is well coated with the dressing and then set aside for a minimum of 30 minutes to marinate.

2. After the steak has had some time to marinate, turn on the grill, and get it preheated to medium-high.

3. Remove the excess dressing and place the steak on the grill.

4. Let the steak grill until it reaches 145 degrees, which will take about 5 minutes on each side.

5. Move the steak to a plate and allow the steak to rest for at least 5 minutes before slicing. Cutting the stake too soon will ruin the steak! Letting it rest is important to a juicy steak.

6. Plate your veggies first as the base of the bowl, then layer the steak over-top. Drizzle with some of the dressing and then serve.

Nutrition:

- Calories 192

- Total Fats 2g

- Carbs: 0.3g

- Protein 42g

- Dietary Fiber: 0g

MEAT

Pork Burgers with Caramelized Onion Rings

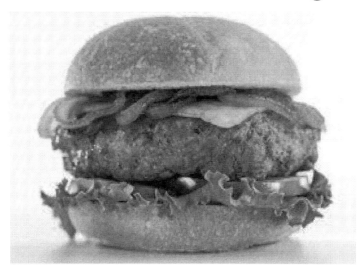

Preparation Time: 5 minutes

Cooking Time:25 minutes

Servings: 8

Ingredients

- 2 lb. ground pork

- Pink salt and chili pepper to taste

- 3 tbsp olive oil

- 1 tbsp butter

- 1 white onion, sliced into rings

- 1 tbsp balsamic vinegar

- 3 drops liquid stevia

- 6 low carb burger buns, halved

- 2 firm tomatoes, sliced into rings

Directions

1. Combine the pork, salt and chili pepper in a bowl and mold out 6 patties.

2. Heat the olive oil in a skillet over medium heat and fry the patties for 4 to 5 minutes on each side until golden brown on the outside. Remove onto a plate and sit for 3 minutes.

3. Melt butter in a skillet over medium heat, sauté onions for 2 minutes, and stir in the balsamic vinegar and liquid stevia.

4. Cook for 30 seconds stirring once or twice until caramelized. In each bun, place a patty, top with some onion rings and 2 tomato rings.

5. Serve the burgers with cheddar cheese dip.

Nutrition:

- Calories 220

- Total Fats 10g

- Carbs: 22g

- Protein 13g

- Dietary Fiber: 1g

Lemon Pork Chops with Buttered Brussels Sprouts

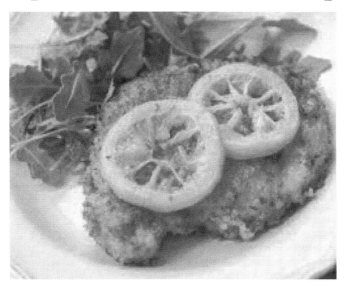

Preparation Time: 5 minutes

Cooking Time: 65 minutes

Servings: 8

Ingredients

- 3 tbsp lemon juice

- 3 cloves garlic, pureed

- 1 tbsp olive oil

- 6 pork loin chops

- 1 tbsp butter

- 1 lb. brussels sprouts, trimmed and halved

- 2 tbsp white wine

- Salt and black pepper to taste

Directions

1. Preheat broiler to 400°F and mix the lemon juice, garlic, salt, black pepper, and oil in a bowl.

2. Brush the pork with the mixture, place in a baking sheet, and cook for 6 minutes on each side until browned. Share into 6 plates and make the side dish.

3. Melt butter in a small wok or pan and cook in brussels sprouts for 5 minutes until tender.

4. Drizzle with white wine, sprinkle with salt and black pepper and cook for another 5 minutes.

5. Ladle brussels sprouts to the side of the chops and serve with a hot sauce.

Nutrition:

- Calories 480

- Total Fats 32g

- Carbs: 17g

- Protein 27g

- Dietary Fiber: 3g

Pork Chops with Cranberry Sauce

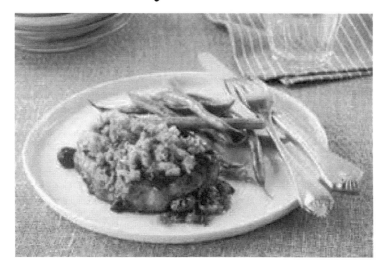

Preparation Time: 5 minutes

Cooking Time: 45 minutes

Servings: 8

Ingredients

- 4 pork chops

- 1 tsp garlic powder

- Salt and black pepper, to taste

- 3 tsp fresh basil, chopped

- A drizzle of olive oil

- 1 shallot, chopped

- 1 cup white wine

- 1 bay leaf

- 2 cups vegetable stock

- Fresh parsley, chopped, for serving

- 2 cups cranberries

- ½ tsp fresh rosemary, chopped

- ½ cup swerve

- Juice of 1 lemon

- 1 cup water

- 1 tsp harissa paste

Directions

1. In a bowl, combine the pork chops with 2 tsp of basil, salt, garlic powder and black pepper. Heat a pan with a drizzle of oil over medium heat, place in the pork and cook until browned; set aside.

2. Stir in the shallot and cook for 2 minutes. Place in the bay leaf and wine and cook for 4 minutes. Pour in juice from ½ lemon, and vegetable stock, and simmer for 5 minutes.

3. Return the pork and cook for 10 minutes. Cover the pan, and place in the oven to bake at 350°F for 2 hours.

4. Set a pan over medium heat, add cranberries, rosemary, harissa paste, water, 1 tsp basil, swerve, and juice from ½ lemon, simmer for 15 minutes.

5. Remove the pork chops from the oven, remove and discard the bay leaf.

6. Split among plates, spread over with the cranberry sauce, sprinkle with parsley to serve.

Nutrition:

- Calories 295

- Fat 15 g

- Carbohydrates 24.4 g

- Sugar 2.2 g

- Protein 17.5 g

- Cholesterol 39 mg

Beef Pot Roast

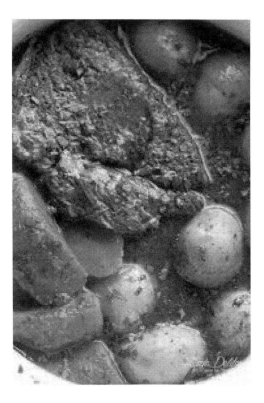

Preparation Time: 10 minutes

Cooking time: 1 hour and 15 minutes

Servings: 6

Ingredients:

- 3½ pounds beef roast
- 4 ounces mushrooms, sliced
- 12 ounces beef stock
- 1 ounce onion powder
- ½ cup olive oil

Directions:

1. In a bowl, mix stock with onion powder, olive oil and stir.

2. Put beef roast in a pan, add mushrooms, stock mixture, cover with aluminum foil, place in an oven at 300°F and bake for 1 hour and 15 minutes.

3. Allow roast to cool, slice, and serve with the gravy on top.

Nutrition:

- Calories 269

- Fat 5.2 g

- Carbohydrates 43.7 g

- Sugar 3.5 g

- Protein 12.4 g

- Cholesterol 59 mg

Beef Zucchini Cups

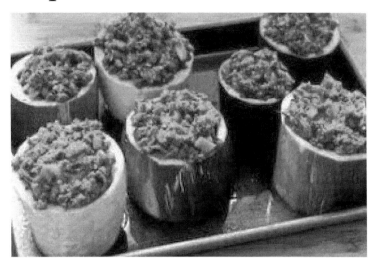

Preparation Time: 10 minutes

Cooking time: 35 minutes

Servings: 6

Ingredients:

- 2 garlic cloves, peeled and minced

- 1 teaspoon cumin

- 1 tablespoon coconut oil

- 1 pound ground beef

- ½ cup onion, chopped

- 1 teaspoon smoked paprika

- Salt and ground black pepper, to taste

- 3 zucchinis, sliced in half lengthwise, and insides scooped out

- ¼ cup fresh cilantro, chopped

- ½ cup cheddar cheese, shredded

- 1½ cups enchilada sauce

- Avocado, chopped, for serving

- Green onions, chopped, for serving

- Tomatoes, cored, and chopped, for serving

Directions:

1. Heat a pan with oil over medium–high heat, add onions, stir, and cook for 2 minutes.

2. Add beef, stir, and brown for a couple of minutes.

3. Add paprika, salt, pepper, cumin, and garlic, stir, and cook for 2 minutes.

4. Place zucchini halves in a baking pan, stuff each with the beef, pour enchilada sauce on top, and sprinkle with cheddar cheese.

5. Bake covered in oven at 350°F for 20 minutes.

6. Uncover pan, sprinkle with the cilantro, and bake for 5 minutes.

7. Sprinkle with avocado, green onions, and tomatoes on top, divide on plates, and serve.

Nutrition:

- Calories 353

- Fat 9.9 g

- Carbohydrates 12.6 g

- Sugar 6.4 g

- Protein 52.5 g

- Cholesterol 286 mg

Ketogenic Beef Sirloin Steak

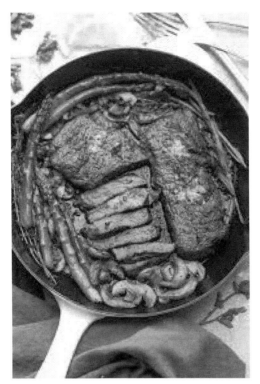

Preparation and Cooking Time: 35 minutes

Servings: 6

Ingredients:

- ½ teaspoon garlic powder

- 3 tablespoons butter

- 1 pound beef top sirloin steaks

- 1 garlic clove, minced

- Salt and freshly ground black pepper, to taste

Directions:

1. Put butter and beef sirloin steaks in a large grill pan.

2. Cook for about 2 minutes on each side to brown the steaks.

3. Add garlic clove, garlic powder, salt, and black pepper and cook for about 15 minutes on each side on medium-high heat.

4. Transfer the steaks in a serving platter and serve hot.

Nutrition:

- Calories 39

- Fat 0.4 g

- Carbohydrates 7.6 g

- Sugar 1.9 g

- Protein 3.2 g

- Cholesterol 0 mg

Beef Fajitas

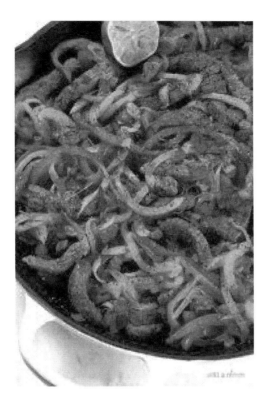

Preparation Time: 20 minutes

Cooking Time: 8 hours

Servings: 6

Ingredients:

- 1 bell pepper, sliced
- 1 tablespoon butter
- 1 pound beef, sliced
- 1 onion, sliced
- 1 tablespoon fajita seasoning

Directions:

1. Place the butter in the bottom of the slow cooker and add onions, fajita seasoning, bell pepper, and beef.

2. Set the slow cooker on LOW and cook for about 8 hours.

3. Dish out the delicious beef fajitas and serve hot.

Nutrition:

- Calories 265
- Fat 10 g
- Carbohydrates 37.9 g
- Sugar 3.2 g
- Protein 7.6 g
- Cholesterol 0 mg

Balsamic Grilled Pork Chops

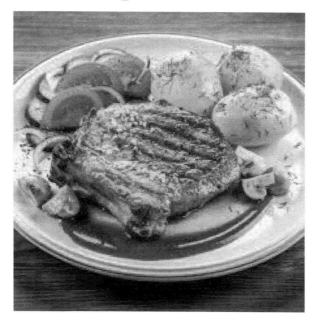

Preparation Time: 10 minutes

Cooking Time:50 minutes

Servings: 6

Ingredients

- 6 pork loin chops, boneless

- 2 tbsp erythritol

- ¼ cup balsamic vinegar

- 3 cloves garlic, minced

- ¼ cup olive oil

- ⅓ tsp salt

- Black pepper to taste

Directions

1. Put the pork in a plastic bag. In a bowl, mix the erythritol, balsamic vinegar, garlic, olive oil, salt, pepper, and pour the sauce over the pork. Seal the bag, shake it, and place in the refrigerator.

2. Marinate the pork for 2 hours. Preheat the grill to medium heat, remove the pork when ready, and grill covered for 10 minutes on each side.

3. Remove and let sit for 4 minutes and serve with parsnip sauté.

Nutrition:

- Calories 169

- Fat 2 g

- Carbohydrates 31.3 g

- Sugar 5.4 g

- Protein 8.7 g

- Cholesterol 0 mg

Pork in White Wine

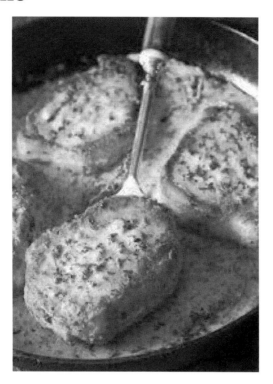

Preparation Time: 10 minutes

Cooking Time:50 minutes

Servings: 6

Ingredients

- 2 tbsp olive oil

- 2 pounds pork stew meat, cubed

- Salt and black pepper, to taste

- 2 tbsp butter

- 4 garlic cloves, minced

- ¾ cup vegetable stock

- ½ cup white wine

- 3 carrots, chopped

- 1 cabbage head, shredded

- ½ cup scallions, chopped

- 1 cup heavy cream

Directions

1. Set a pan over medium heat and warm butter and oil. Sear the pork until brown. Add garlic, scallions, and carrots; sauté for 5 minutes.

2. Pour in the cabbage, stock, and wine, and bring to a boil. Reduce the heat and cook for 1 hour covered.

3. Add in heavy cream as you stir for 1 minute, adjust seasonings and serve.

Nutrition:

- Calories 157

- Fat 9.5g

- Carb 9.3g

- Protein 12.4g

- Sugars 3.2g

Stuffed Pork with Red Cabbage Salad

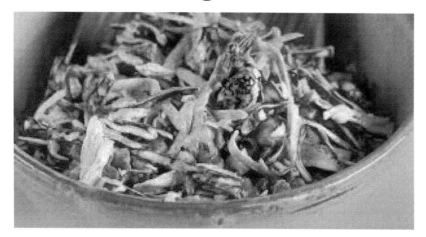

Preparation Time: 10 minutes

Cooking Time:60 minutes

Servings: 6

Ingredients

- Zest and juice from 2 limes

- 2 garlic cloves, minced

- ¾ cup olive oil

- 1 cup fresh cilantro, chopped

- 1 cup fresh mint, chopped

- 1 tsp dried oregano

- Salt and black pepper, to taste

- 2 tsp cumin

- 4 pork loin steaks

- 2 pickles, chopped

- 4 ham slices

- 6 Swiss cheese slices

- 2 tbsp mustard

- For the Salad

- 1 head red cabbage, shredded

- 2 tbsp vinegar

- 3 tbsp olive oil

- Salt to taste

Directions

1. In a food processor, blitz the lime zest, oil, oregano, black pepper, cumin, cilantro, lime juice, garlic, mint, and salt. Rub the steaks with the mixture and toss well to coat; set aside for some hours in the fridge.

2. Arrange the steaks on a working surface, split the pickles, mustard, cheese, and ham on them, roll, and secure with toothpicks.

3. Heat a pan over medium heat, add in the pork rolls, cook each side for 2 minutes and remove to a baking sheet. Bake in the oven at 350°F for 25 minutes.

4. Prepare the red cabbage salad by mixing all salad ingredients and serve with the meat.

Nutrition:

- Calories 109

- Fat 7.1g

- Carbs 8g

- Protein 2.8g

- Sugars 2.8g

Spicy Mesquite Pork Ribs

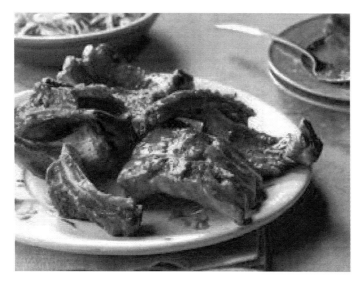

Preparation Time: 10 minutes

Cooking Time: 30 minutes

Servings: 6

Ingredients

- 3 racks pork ribs, silver lining removed
- 2 cups sugar-free BBQ sauce
- 2 tbsp erythritol
- 2 tsp chili powder
- 2 tsp cumin powder
- 2 tsp onion powder
- 2 tsp smoked paprika
- 2 tsp garlic powder
- Salt and black pepper to taste
- 1 tsp mustard powder

Directions

1. Preheat a smoker to 400°F using mesquite wood to create flavor in the smoker.

2. In a bowl, mix the erythritol, chili powder, cumin powder, black pepper, onion powder, smoked paprika, garlic powder, salt, and mustard powder. Rub the ribs and let marinate for 30 minutes.

3. Place on the grill grate and cook at reduced heat of 225°F for 4 hours.

4. Flip the ribs after and continue cooking for 4 hours. Brush the ribs with BBQ sauce on both sides and sear them in increased heat for 3 minutes per side.

5. Remove and let sit for 4 minutes before slicing. Serve with red cabbage coleslaw.

Nutrition:

- Calories 176
- Fat 13.7g
- Carbs 9g
- Protein 7g
- Sugars 1.5g

Paprika Pork Chops

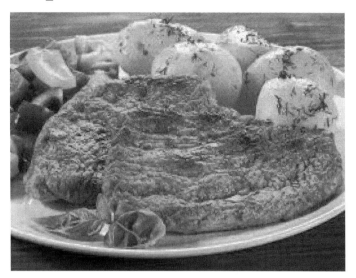

Preparation Time: 10 minutes

Cooking Time: 20 minutes

Servings: 6

Ingredients

- 4 pork chops
- Salt and black pepper, to taste
- 3 tbsp paprika
- ¾ cup cumin powder
- 1 tsp chili powder

Directions

1. In a bowl, combine the paprika with black pepper, cumin, salt, and chili. Place in the pork chops and rub them well.

2. Heat a grill over medium temperature, add in the pork chops, cook for 5 minutes, flip, and cook for 5 minutes. Serve with steamed veggies.

Nutrition: Calories 314 - Fat: 17.4g - Carbo: 39.3g - Dietary Fiber: 3.7g - Protein: 7.3g

Beef Cauliflower Curry

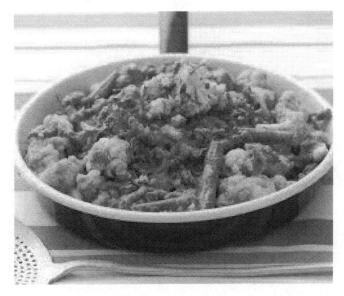

Preparation Time: 10 minutes

Cooking Time: 50 minutes

Servings: 6

Ingredients

- 1 tbsp olive oil

- 1 ½ lb. ground beef

- 1 tbsp ginger-garlic paste

- 1 tsp garam masala

- 1 (7 oz) can whole tomatoes

- 1 head cauliflower, cut into florets

- Pink salt and chili pepper to taste

- ¼ cup water

Directions

3. Heat oil in a saucepan over medium heat, add the beef, ginger-garlic paste and season with garam masala.

4. Cook for 5 minutes while breaking any lumps.

5. Stir in the tomatoes and cauliflower, season with salt and chili pepper, and cook covered for 6 minutes.

6. Add the water and bring to a boil over medium heat for 10 minutes or until the water has reduced by half.

7. Adjust taste with salt. Spoon the curry into serving bowls and serve with shirataki rice.

Nutrition:

- Calories 150

- Fat: 14.4g

- Carbohydrates: 4.7g

- Dietary Fiber: 1.4g

- Protein: 4.4g

Easy Zucchini Beef Lasagna

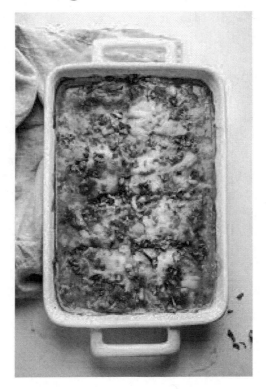

Preparation Time: 10 minutes

Cooking Time: 20 minutes

Servings: 6

Ingredients

- 1 lb. ground beef

- 2 large zucchinis, sliced lengthwise

- 3 cloves garlic

- 1 medium white onion, finely chopped

- 3 tomatoes, chopped

- Salt and black pepper to taste

- 2 tsp sweet paprika

- 1 tsp dried thyme

- 1 tsp dried basil

- 1 cup shredded mozzarella cheese

- 1 tbsp olive oil

- Cooking spray

Directions

1. Preheat the oven to 370°F and lightly grease a baking dish with cooking spray.

2. Heat the olive oil in a skillet and cook the beef for 4 minutes while breaking any lumps as you stir. Top with onion, garlic, tomatoes, salt, paprika, and pepper. Stir and continue cooking for 5 minutes.

3. Then, lay ⅓ of the zucchini slices in the baking dish. Top with ⅓ of the beef mixture and repeat the layering process two more times with the same quantities. Season with basil and thyme.

4. Finally, sprinkle the mozzarella cheese on top and tuck the baking dish in the oven. Bake for 35 minutes. Remove the lasagna and let it rest for 10 minutes before serving.

Beefy and Cheesy Green Chile Bake

Put this dish on the dinner table and just let everyone decide.

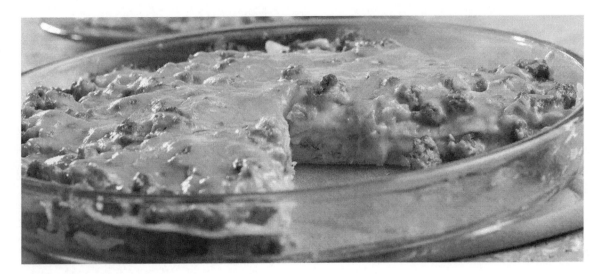

Preparation Time: 20 minutes

Cooking Time: 40 minutes

Servings: 8

Ingredients:

- 1 large can + 1 4 oz. can Green Chilies

- 4 tsp Olive Oil

- 1 lb. Ground Beef

- Salt to taste

- Black Pepper to taste

- 4 cups Mexican Cheese

- 1 Onion

- 5 Eggs

- ½ cup Sour Cream

- ½ tsp Ground Cumin

- ½ tsp Chili Powder

Directions

1. Cook the ground beef on a medium flame until brown. Add salt and pepper to taste.

2. Cook the onion and green chilies for 2-3 minutes. Afterward, add in the ground beef to this pan.

3. Beat the eggs in a bowl and add in the cumin, chili powder, and sour cream. Whisk together until well combined.

4. Wash some green chilies in a colander and split them open to remove the seeds. Place these chilies in a layer in a casserole dish followed by a layer of ground beef, cheese and the egg mixture.

5. Bake the assembly in a preheated oven at 400 F for 15 minutes.

6. Serve with toppings of your choice.

Nutrition:

- Calories 111

- Fat: 4.3g

- Carbohydrates: 9.8g

- Dietary Fiber: 4.1g

- Protein: 9.83g

Grilled Sirloin Steak with Sauce Diane

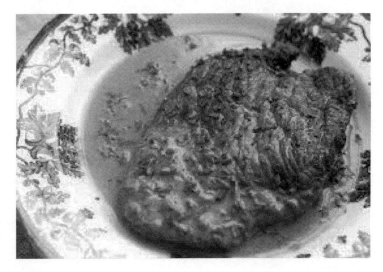

Preparation Time: 10 minutes

Cooking Time:50 minutes

Servings: 6

Ingredients

- Sirloin Steak

- 1 ½ lb. sirloin steak

- Salt and black pepper to taste

- 1 tsp olive oil

- Sauce Diane

- 1 tbsp olive oil

- 1 clove garlic, minced

- 1 cup sliced porcini mushrooms

- 1 small onion, finely diced

- 2 tbsp butter

- 1 tbsp Dijon mustard

- 2 tbsp Worcestershire sauce

- ¼ cup whiskey

- 2 cups double cream

- Salt and black pepper to taste

Directions

1. Put a grill pan over high heat and as it heats, brush the steak with oil, sprinkle with salt and pepper, and rub the seasoning into the meat with your hands.

2. Cook the steak in the pan for 4 minutes on each side for medium rare and transfer to a chopping board to rest for 4 minutes before slicing. Reserve the juice.

3. Heat the oil in a frying pan over medium heat and sauté the onion for 3 minutes. Add the butter, garlic, and mushrooms, and cook for 2 minutes.

4. Add the Worcestershire sauce, the reserved juice, and mustard. Stir and cook for 1 minute.

5. Pour in the whiskey and cook further 1 minute until the sauce reduces by half. Swirl the pan and add the cream. Let it simmer to thicken for about 3 minutes. Adjust the taste with salt and pepper.

6. Spoon the sauce over the steaks slices and serve with celeriac mash.

Nutrition:

- Calories 172

- Fat 9.9 g

- Carbohydrates 20.8 g

- Sugar 9.7 g

- Protein 4.1 g

- Cholesterol 0 mg

Italian Beef Ragout

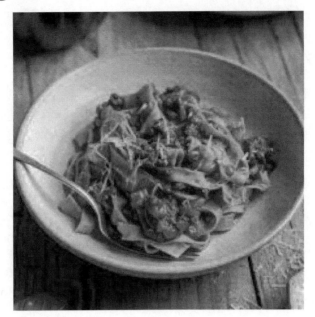

Preparation Time: 10 minutes

Cooking Time:30 minutes

Servings: 6

Ingredients

- 1 lb. chuck steak, trimmed and cubed

- 2 tbsp olive oil

- Salt and black pepper to taste

- 2 tbsp almond flour

- 1 medium onion, diced

- ½ cup dry white wine

- 1 red bell pepper, seeded and diced

- 2 tsp Worcestershire sauce

- 4 oz tomato puree

- 3 tsp smoked paprika

- 1 cup beef broth

- Thyme leaves to garnish

Directions

1. First, lightly dredge the meat in the almond flour and set aside. Place a large skillet over medium heat, add 1 tablespoon of oil to heat and then sauté the onion, and bell pepper for 3 minutes.

2. Stir in the paprika and add the remaining olive oil.

3. Add the beef and cook for 10 minutes in total while turning them halfway. Stir in white wine, let it reduce by half, about 3 minutes, and add Worcestershire sauce, tomato puree, and beef broth.

4. Let the mixture boil for 2 minutes, then reduce the heat to lowest and let simmer for 1 ½ hours; stirring now and then.

5. Adjust the taste and dish the ragout. Serve garnished with thyme leaves

BBQ Beef Burritos

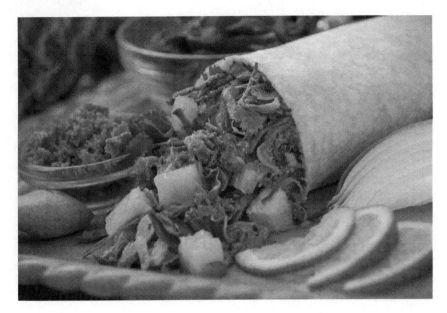

Preparation Time: 35 minutes

Cooking Time: 8 hours

Servings: 4

Ingredients:

- 2 lb. top sirloin steak

- ½ t. black pepper

- 1 t. of Ground chipotle pepper – optional

- 1 t. of Cinnamon

- 2 t. of Sea salt

- 2 t. of Garlic powder

- 4 minced garlic cloves

- ½ white onion

- 2 bay leaves

- 1 c. of Chicken broth

- 1 c. of BBQ sauce – your favorite

- Assembly Ingredients:

- 1 ½ c. coleslaw mix

- 8 low-carb wraps

- ½ c. mayonnaise

Directions:

1. Pat the steak dry using some paper towels. Score with a sharp knife along the sides. Combine the seasonings and sprinkle on the meat.

2. Roughly chop the onion and mince the garlic and add to the crockpot. Pour in the broth. Add the steak and bay leaf. Secure the lid and cook eight hours on the low setting

3. When done, remove the steak and drain the juices. Arrange the beef, garlic, and onion back into the cooker and shred. Pour in the barbecue sauce and mix well.

4. Assemble the burritos using the beef fixings, a bit of slaw, and a dab of mayo.

Nutrition:

- Calories 153

- Total Fat: 6.7g

- Carbs: 19.7g

- Sugars: 5.4g

- Protein: 5g

Beef Cotija Cheeseburger

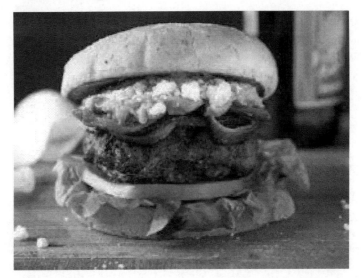

Preparation Time: 10 minutes

Cooking Time: 20 minutes

Servings: 6

- **Ingredients**

- 1 lb. ground beef

- 1 tsp dried parsley

- ½ tsp Worcestershire sauce

- Salt and black pepper to taste

- 1 cup cotija cheese, shredded

- 4 low carb buns, halved

Directions

1. Preheat a grill to 400°F and grease the grate with cooking spray.

2. Mix the beef, parsley, Worcestershire sauce, salt, and black pepper with your hands until evenly combined. Make medium sized patties out of the mixture, about 4 patties. Cook on the grill for 7 minutes one side to be cooked through and no longer pink.

3. Flip the patties and top with cheese. Cook for 7 minutes, until the cheese melts.

4. Remove the patties and sandwich into two halves of a bun each. Serve with a tomato dipping sauce and zucchini fries.

Nutrition:

- Calories 202
- Total Fat: 5.2g
- Carbs: 40.6g
- Sugars: 9g
- Protein: 3.6g

Warm Rump Steak Salad

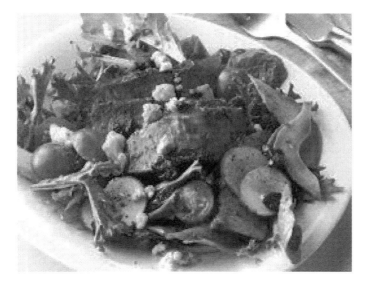

Preparation Time: 10 minutes

Cooking Time:50 minutes

Servings: 6

Ingredients

- ½ lb. rump steak, excess fat trimmed
- 3 green onions, sliced

- 3 tomatoes, sliced

- 1 cup green beans, steamed and sliced

- 2 kohlrabi, peeled and chopped

- ½ cup water

- 2 cups mixed salad greens

- Salt and black pepper to season

- Salad Dressing

- 2 tsp Dijon mustard

- 1 tsp erythritol

- Salt and black pepper to taste

- 3 tbsp olive oil + extra for drizzling

- 1 tbsp red wine vinegar

Directions

1. Preheat the oven to 400°F. Place the kohlrabi on a baking sheet, drizzle with olive oil and bake in the oven for 25 minutes. After cooking, remove, and set aside to cool.

2. In a bowl, mix the Dijon mustard, erythritol, salt, black pepper, vinegar, and olive oil. Set aside.

3. Then, preheat a grill pan over high heat while you season the meat with salt and black pepper. Place the steak in the pan and brown on both sides for 4 minutes each. Remove to rest on a chopping board for 4 more minutes before slicing thinly.

4. In a salad bowl, add green onions, tomatoes, green beans, kohlrabi, salad greens, and steak slices.

5. Drizzle the dressing over and toss with two spoons. Serve the steak salad warm with chunks of low carb bread.

Nutrition: Calories 286 - Total Fat: 8.6g - Carbs: 44.6g - Sugars: 6.7g - Protein: 9.3g

Beef with Dilled Yogurt

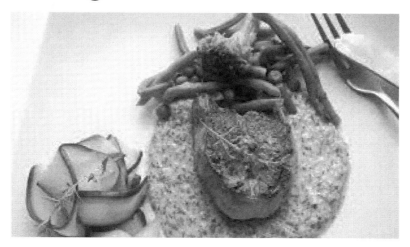

Preparation Time: 10 minutes

Cooking Time: 40 minutes

Servings: 6

Ingredients

- ¼ cup almond milk

- 2 pounds ground beef

- 1 onion, grated

- 5 zero carb bread slices, torn

- 1 egg, whisked

- ¼ cup fresh parsley, chopped

- Salt and black pepper, to taste

- 2 garlic cloves, minced

- ¼ cup fresh mint, chopped

- 2 ½ tsp dried oregano

- ¼ cup olive oil

- 1 cup cherry tomatoes, halved

- 1 cucumber, sliced

- 1 cup baby spinach

- 1½ tbsp lemon juice

- 1 cup dilled Greek yogurt

Directions

1. Place the torn bread in a bowl, add in the milk, and set aside for 3 minutes. Squeeze the bread, chop, and place into a bowl.

2. Stir in the beef, salt, mint, onion, parsley, pepper, egg, oregano, and garlic.

3. Form balls out of this mixture and place on a working surface. Set a pan over medium heat and warm half of the oil; fry the meatballs for 8 minutes.

4. Flip occasionally and set aside in a tray.

5. In a salad plate, combine the spinach with the cherry tomatoes and cucumber.

6. Mix in the remaining oil, lemon juice, black pepper, and salt. Spread dilled yogurt over, and top with meatballs to serve.

Nutrition:

- Calories 87

- Total Fat: 5.2g

- Carbs: 8.6g

- Sugars: 3.9g

- Protein: 3.9g

Beef Stovies

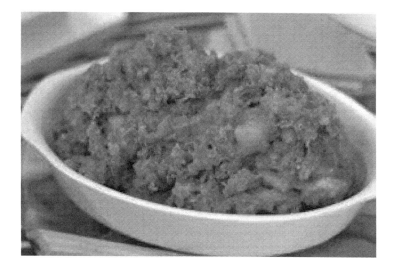

Preparation Time: 10 minutes

Cooking Time:34 minutes

Servings: 6

Ingredients

- 1 lb. ground beef

- 1 large onion, chopped

- 6 parsnips, peeled and chopped

- 1 large carrot, chopped

- 1 tbsp olive oil

- 1 clove garlic, minced

- Salt and black pepper to taste

- 1 cup chicken broth

- ¼ tsp allspice

- 2 tsp rosemary leaves

- 1 tbsp sugar-free Worcestershire sauce

- ½ small cabbage, shredded

Directions

1. Heat the oil in a skillet over medium heat and cook the beef for 4 minutes. Season with salt and black pepper, and occasionally stir while breaking the lumps in it.

2. Add in the onion, garlic, carrot, rosemary, and parsnips. Stir and cook for a minute, and pour the chicken broth, allspice, and Worcestershire sauce in it. Stir the mixture and cook the ingredients on low heat for 40 minutes.

3. Stir in the cabbage, season with salt and black pepper, and cook further for 2 minutes.

4. After, turn the heat off, plate the stovies, and serve with wilted spinach and collards.

Nutrition:

- Calories 174

- Total Fat: 10.4g

- Carbs: 17.1g

- Sugars: 3.9g

- Protein: 8.5g

Beef with Grilled Vegetables

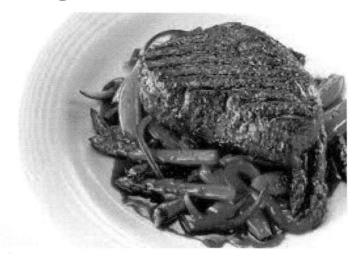

Preparation Time: 10 minutes

Cooking Time:30 minutes

Servings: 6

Ingredients

- 4 sirloin steaks

- Salt and black pepper to taste

- 4 tbsp olive oil

- 3 tbsp balsamic vinegar

- Vegetables

- ½ lb. asparagus, trimmed

- 1 cup green beans

- 1 cup snow peas

- 1 red bell peppers, seeded, cut into strips

- 1 orange bell peppers, seeded, cut into strips

- 1 medium red onion, quartered

Directions

1. Set the grill pan over high heat.

2. Grab 2 separate bowls; put the beef in one and the vegetables in another. Mix salt, pepper, olive oil, and balsamic vinegar in a small bowl, and pour half of the mixture over the beef and the other half over the vegetables.

3. Coat the ingredients in both bowls with the sauce and cook the beef first.

4. Place the steaks in the grill pan and sear both sides for 2 minutes each, then continue cooking for 6 minutes on each side. When done, remove the beef onto a plate; set aside.

5. Pour the vegetables and marinade in the pan; and cook for 5 minutes, turning once. Share the vegetables into plates.

6. Top with each piece of beef, the sauce from the pan, and serve with a rutabaga mash.

Nutrition:

- Calories 178

- Fat 10.7g

- Carbs 18.2g

- Protein 5.9g

- Sugars 6g

Ribeye Steak with Shitake Mushrooms

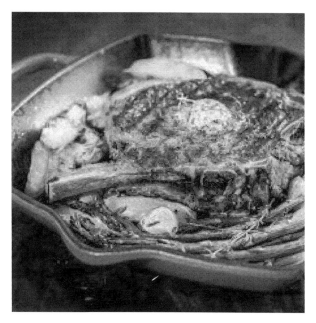

Preparation Time: 10 minutes

Cooking Time:40 minutes

Servings: 6

Ingredients

- 6 ounces ribeye steak

- 2 tbsp butter

- 1 tsp olive oil

- ½ cup shitake mushrooms, sliced

- Salt and black pepper, to taste

Directions

1. Heat the olive oil in a pan over medium heat. Rub the steak with salt and black pepper and cook about 4 minutes per side; set aside.

2. Melt the butter in the pan and cook the shitakes for 4 minutes. Pour the butter and mushrooms over the steak to serve.

Nutrition: Calories 98 - Fat 3.6 g - Carbo 14.5g - Sugar 0g - Protein 3g – Cholesterol 0 mg

POULTRY

Spanish Chicken

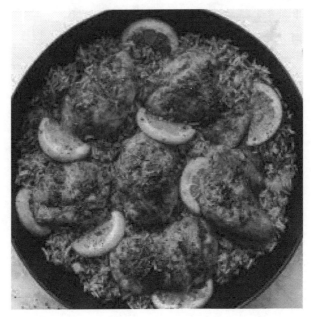

Preparation Time: 10 minutes

Cooking Time:50 minutes

Servings: 6

Ingredients

- 1/2 cup mushrooms, chopped

- 1 pound chorizo sausages, chopped

- 2 tbsp avocado oil

- 4 cherry peppers, chopped

- 1 red bell pepper, seeded, chopped

- 1 onion, peeled and sliced

- 2 tbsp garlic, minced

- 2 cups tomatoes, chopped

- 4 chicken thighs

- Salt and black pepper, to taste

- ½ cup chicken stock

- 1 tsp turmeric

- 1 tbsp vinegar

- 2 tsp dried oregano

- Fresh parsley, chopped, for serving

Directions

1. Set a pan over medium heat and warm half of the avocado oil, stir in the chorizo sausages, and cook for 5-6 minutes until browned; remove to a bowl. Heat the rest of the oil, place in the chicken thighs, and apply pepper and salt for seasoning.

2. Cook each side for 3 minutes and set aside on a bowl.

3. In the same pan, add the onion, bell pepper, cherry peppers, and mushrooms, and cook for 4 minutes.

4. Stir in the garlic and cook for 2 minutes. Pour in the stock, turmeric, salt, tomatoes, pepper, vinegar, and oregano.

5. Stir in the chorizo sausages and chicken, place everything to the oven at 400°F, and bake for 30 minutes.

6. Ladle into serving bowls and garnish with chopped parsley to serve.

Nutrition:

- Calories 348

- Fat 38.7g

- Carbs 3.2g

- Protein 0.6g

- Sugars 1.7g

Cheesy Chicken Bake with Zucchini

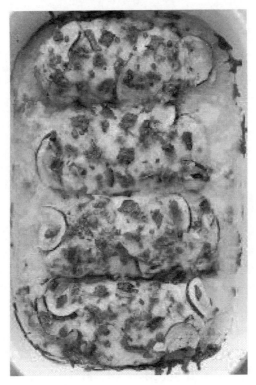

Preparation Time: 10 minutes

Cooking Time:70 minutes

Servings: 6

Ingredients

- 2 lb. chicken breasts, cubed

- 1 tbsp butter

- 1 cup green bell peppers, sliced

- 1 cup yellow onions, sliced

- 1 zucchini, cubed

- 2 garlic cloves, divided

- 2 tsp Italian seasoning

- ½ tsp salt

- ½ tsp black pepper

- 8 oz cream cheese, softened

- ½ cup mayonnaise

- 2 tbsp Worcestershire sauce (sugar-free)

- 2 cups cheddar cheese, shredded

Directions

1. Set oven to 370°F and grease and line a baking dish.

2. Set a pan over medium heat. Place in the butter and let melt, then add in the chicken. Cook until lightly browned, about 5 minutes.

3. Place in onions, zucchini, black pepper, garlic, bell peppers, salt, and 1 tsp of Italian seasoning. Cook until tender and set aside.

4. In a bowl, mix cream cheese, garlic, remaining seasoning, mayonnaise, and Worcestershire sauce.

5. Stir in meat and sauteed vegetables.

6. Place the mixture into the prepared baking dish, sprinkle with the shredded cheddar cheese and insert into the oven.

7. Cook until browned for 30 minutes.

Nutrition:

- Calories 308

- Fat 28.3g

- Carbs 4.5g

- Protein 12.3g

- Sugars 1.4g

Chicken Skewers with Celery Fries

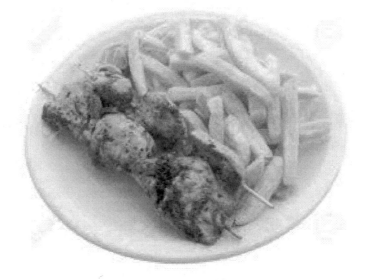

Preparation Time: 10 minutes

Cooking Time:20 minutes

Servings: 6

Ingredients

- 2 chicken breasts

- ½ tsp salt

- ¼ tsp ground black pepper

- 2 tbsp olive oil

- 1/4 cup chicken broth

- For the fries

- 1 lb. celery root

- 2 tbsp olive oil

- ½ tsp salt

- ¼ tsp ground black pepper

Directions

1. Set oven to 400°F. Grease and line a baking sheet. In a bowl, mix oil, spices and the chicken; set in the fridge for 10 minutes while covered.

2. Peel and chop celery root to form fry shapes and place into a separate bowl. Apply oil to coat and add pepper and salt for seasoning.

3. Arrange to the baking tray in an even layer and bake for 10 minutes.

4. Take the chicken from the refrigerator and thread onto the skewers.

5. Place over the celery, pour in the chicken broth, then set in the oven for 30 minutes. Serve with lemon wedges.

Nutrition:

- Calories 144

- Fat 11.4g

- Carbs 9.2g

- Protein 3.3g

- Sugars 3.5g

One Pot Chicken with Mushrooms

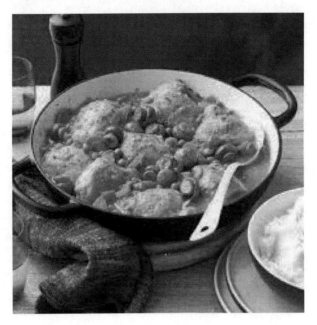

Preparation Time: 10 minutes

Cooking Time: 50 minutes

Servings: 6

Ingredients

- 2 cups sliced mushrooms

- ½ tsp onion powder

- ½ tsp garlic powder

- ¼ cup butter

- 1 tsp Dijon mustard

- 1 tbsp tarragon, chopped

- 2 pounds chicken thighs

- Salt and black pepper, to taste

Directions

1. Season the thighs with salt, pepper, garlic, and onion powder. Melt the butter in a skillet and cook the chicken until browned; set aside.

2. Add mushrooms to the same fat and cook for about 5 minutes.

3. Stir in Dijon mustard and ½ cup of water.

4. Return the chicken to the skillet. Season to taste with salt and pepper, reduce the heat and cover, and let simmer for 15 minutes.

5. Stir in tarragon. Serve warm.

Nutrition:

- Calories 141
- Fat 11.1g
- Carbs 9.1g
- Protein 2.2g
- Sugars 4.2g

Chicken in Creamy Tomato Sauce

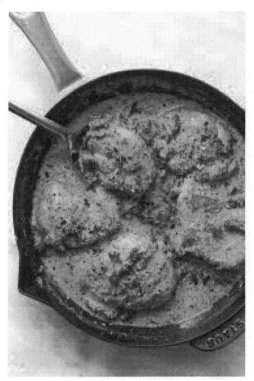

Preparation Time: 10 minutes

Cooking Time:50 minutes

Servings: 6

Ingredients

- 2 tbsp butter

- 6 chicken thighs

- Pink salt and black pepper to taste

- 14 oz canned tomato sauce

- 2 tsp Italian seasoning

- ½ cup heavy cream

- 1 cup shredded Parmesan cheese

- Parmesan cheese to garnish.

Directions

1. In a saucepan, melt the butter over medium heat, season the chicken with salt and black pepper, and cook for 5 minutes on each side to brown. Place the chicken.

2. Pour the tomato sauce and Italian seasoning in the pan and cook covered for 8 minutes.

3. Adjust the taste with salt and black pepper and stir in the heavy cream and Parmesan cheese.

4. Once the cheese has melted, return the chicken to the pot, and simmer for 4 minutes.

5. Dish the chicken with sauce, garnish with more Parmesan cheese, and serve with zoodles.

Nutrition:

- Calories 243
- Fat: 8.3g
- Carbohydrates: 33.23g
- Dietary Fiber: 11.96g
- Protein: 13.4g

Sticky Cranberry Chicken Wings

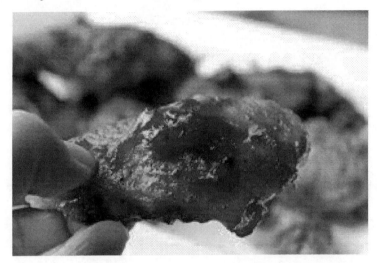

Preparation Time: 10 minutes

Cooking Time:50 minutes

Servings: 6

Ingredients

- 2 lb. chicken wings

- 4 tbsp unsweetened cranberry puree

- 2 tbsp olive oil

- Salt to taste

- Sweet chili sauce to taste

- Lemon juice from 1 lemon

Directions

1. Preheat oven to 400°F. In a bowl, mix cranberry puree, olive oil, salt, sweet chili sauce, and lemon juice.

2. Add in the wings and toss to coat. Place the chicken under the broiler, and cook for 45 minutes, turning once halfway.

3. Remove the chicken after and serve warm with a cranberry and cheese dipping sauce.

Nutrition: Calories 106 – Fat 7.7g – Carbs 7g – Protein 3.5g – Sugars 1.7g

Grilled Paprika Chicken with Steamed Broccoli

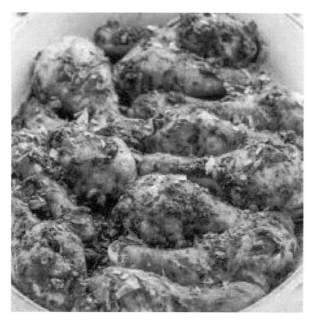

Preparation Time: 10 minutes

Cooking Time:30 minutes

Servings: 6

Ingredients

- 3 tbsp smoked paprika

- Salt and black pepper to taste

- 2 tsp garlic powder

- 1 tbsp olive oil

- 6 chicken breasts

- 1 head broccoli, cut into florets

Directions

1. Place broccoli florets onto the steamer basket over the boiling water; steam approximately 8 minutes or until crisp-tender.

2. Set aside. Grease grill grate with cooking spray and preheat to 400°F.

3. Combine paprika, salt, black pepper, and garlic powder in a bowl.

4. Brush chicken with olive oil and sprinkle spice mixture over and massage with hands.

5. Grill chicken for 7 minutes per side until well-cooked, and plate. Serve warm with steamed broccoli.

Nutrition:

- Calories 74
- Fat 6.1g
- Carbs 3.5g
- Protein 1.7g
- Sugars 1.5g

Chicken with Anchovy Tapenade

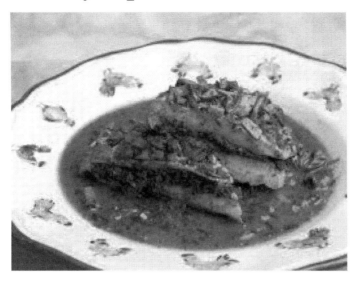

Preparation Time: 10 minutes

Cooking Time: 30 minutes

Servings: 6

Ingredients

- 1 chicken breast, cut into 4 pieces

- 2 tbsp coconut oil

- 3 garlic cloves, crushed

- For the tapenade

- 1 cup black olives, pitted

- 1 oz anchovy fillets, rinsed

- 1 garlic clove, crushed

- Salt and ground black pepper, to taste

- 2 tbsp olive oil

- ¼ cup fresh basil, chopped

- 1 tbsp lemon juice

Directions

1. Using a food processor, combine the olives, salt, olive oil, basil, lemon juice, anchovy, and black pepper, blend well.

2. Set a pan over medium heat and warm coconut oil, stir in the garlic, and sauté for 2 minutes.

3. Place in the chicken pieces and cook each side for 4 minutes.

4. Split the chicken among plates and apply a topping of the anchovy tapenade.

Nutrition:

- Calories 89

- Fat 7.1g

- Carbs 6.4g

- Protein 0.7g

- Sugars 3.1g

Bacon & Cheese Chicken

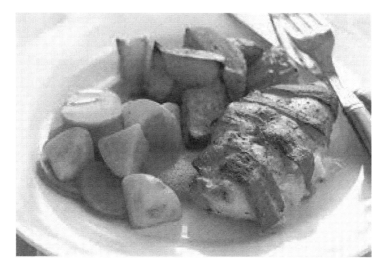

Preparation Time: 10 minutes

Cooking Time: 30 minutes

Servings: 6

Ingredients

- 4 bacon strips

- 4 chicken breasts

- 3 green onions, chopped

- 4 ounces ranch dressing

- 1 ounce coconut aminos

- 2 tbsp coconut oil

- 4 oz Monterey Jack cheese, grated

Directions

1. Set a pan over high heat and warm the oil. Place in the chicken breasts, cook for 7 minutes, then flip to the other side Cooking for an additional 7 minutes.

2. Set another pan over medium heat, place in the bacon, cook until crispy, remove to paper towels, drain the grease, and crumble.

3. Add the chicken breast to a baking dish. Place the green onions, coconut aminos, cheese, and crumbled bacon on top, set in an oven, turn on the broiler, and cook for 5 minutes at high temperature.

4. Split among serving plates and serve.

Nutrition:

- Calories 278

- Fat: 21.5g

- Carbohydrates: 15.3g

- Dietary Fiber: 4.3g

- Protein: 8.4g

Fried Chicken with Paprika Sauce

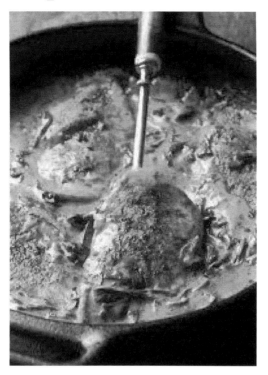

Preparation Time: 10 minutes

Cooking time: 20 minutes

Servings: 6

Ingredients:

- 1 tablespoon coconut oil

- 3½ pounds chicken breasts

- 1 cup chicken stock

- 1¼ cups onion, peeled and chopped

- 1 tablespoon lime juice

- ¼ cup coconut milk

- 2 teaspoons paprika

- 1 teaspoon red pepper flakes

- 2 tablespoons green onions, chopped

- Salt and ground black pepper, to taste

Directions:

1. Heat a pan with oil over medium–high heat, add chicken, cook for 2 minutes on each side, transfer to a plate, and set aside.

2. Reduce heat to medium, add onions to the pan, and cook for 4 minutes.

3. Add stock, coconut milk, pepper flakes, paprika, lime juice, salt, pepper, and stir well.

4. Return chicken to pan, add more salt, pepper, cover the pan, and cook for 15 minutes.

5. Divide on plates and serve.

Nutrition:

- Calories 659

- Fat 33.8 g

- Carbohydrates 73.9 g

- Sugar 17.7 g

- Protein 23.1 g

- Cholesterol 0 mg

Rosemary Balsamic Chicken Liver Pate

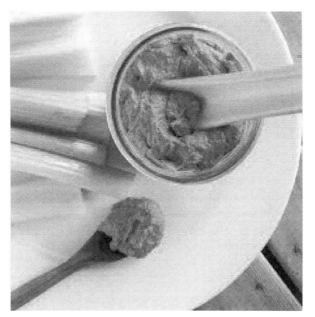

Preparation and Cooking Time: 12-24 hours to marinate the liver and 25 minutes

Ingredients:

Servings: 6

- 1 pound of chicken liver
- 1 cup of chopped leek, green parts
- 1 tablespoon of apple cider vinegar
- 2-3 tablespoon of balsamic vinegar
- ¼ cup of coconut oil
- 1 sprig of fresh rosemary (removed from the stem)
- 1 teaspoon of freshly ground pepper
- ½ teaspoon of sea salt
- filtered water

Directions:

1. (Add enough water to the tablespoon of apple cider vinegar so that the solution completely covers the liver)

2. After marinating, drain the liver and place it in a cast iron pan along with coconut oil, rosemary, leeks, and salt.

3. Cover and cook on medium-low heat for 10 minutes.

4. Remove from heat and set aside for 5 minutes.

5. Transfer the liver and juices to your blender.

6. Add balsamic vinegar and ground pepper.

7. Blend until very smooth.

8. Spoon the mixture into a shallow sealable container.

9. Seal container and store in the fridge for 2 to 3 days before serving.

Nutrition:

- Calories 349
- Fat 14.4 g
- Carbohydrates 40.8 g
- Sugar 3.3 g
- Protein 14.1 g
- Cholesterol 41 mg

Chicken Fajitas

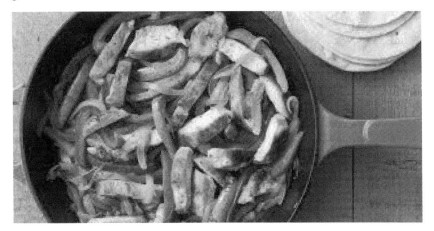

Preparation Time: 10 minutes

Cooking time: 15 minutes

Servings: 6

Ingredients:

- 2 pounds chicken breasts, skinless, boneless, and cut into strips
- 1 teaspoon garlic powder
- 1 teaspoon chili powder
- 2 teaspoons cumin
- 2 tablespoons lime juice
- Salt and ground black pepper, to taste
- 1 teaspoon sweet paprika
- 2 tablespoons coconut oil
- 1 teaspoon coriander
- 1 green bell pepper, seeded and sliced
- 1 red bell pepper, seeded and sliced
- 1 onion, peeled and sliced

- 1 tablespoon fresh cilantro, chopped

- 1 avocado, pitted, peeled, and sliced

- 2 limes, cut into wedges

Directions:

1. In a bowl, mix lime juice with chili powder, cumin, salt, pepper, garlic powder, paprika, coriander, and stir.

2. Add chicken pieces and toss to coat well.

3. Heat a pan with half of the oil over medium–high heat, add chicken, cook for 3 minutes on each side, and transfer to a bowl.

4. Heat the pan with remaining oil over medium heat, add onion and bell peppers, stir, and cook for 6 minutes.

5. Return chicken to pan, add more salt, pepper, stir, and divide on plates.

6. Top with avocado, lime wedges, cilantro, and serve.

Nutrition:

- Calories 30

- Fat 0.2 g

- Carbohydrates 5.1 g

- Sugar 0.1 g

- Protein 2.2 g

- Cholesterol 0 mg

Rainbow Stir Fry

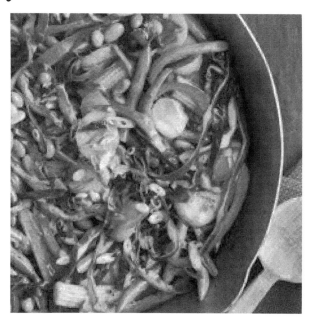

Preparation and Cooking Time: 15-20 minutes

Servings: 6

Ingredients:

- 2 cup cooked chicken
- 6 peeled carrots
- ½ small diced onion
- 2 cloves of minced garlic
- 3-4 tablespoon of coconut aminos
- 1-2 cups of green beans
- ¼ cup of real butter
- sea salt
- pepper

Directions:

1. In a large pan, sauté the diced onion in butter for 5 minutes.

2. Add a bit of sea salt.

3. Add garlic and cook for another minute.

4. Add green beans, carrots, coconut aminos, and chicken. Cook on medium heat until the vegetables are cooked through.

5. Add salt and pepper to taste.

Nutrition:

- Calories 61

- Fat 1.6 g

- Carbohydrates 11.2 g

- Sugar 5.6 g

- Protein 0.9 g

- Cholesterol 4 mg

Skillet Chicken and Mushrooms

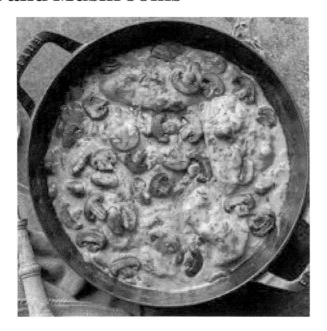

Preparation Time: 10 minutes

Cooking time: 30 minutes

Servings: 6

Ingredients:

- 4 chicken thighs

- 2 cups mushrooms, sliced

- ¼ cup butter

- Salt and ground black pepper, to taste

- ½ teaspoon onion powder

- ½ teaspoon garlic powder

- ½ cup water

- 1 teaspoon Dijon mustard

- 1 tablespoon fresh tarragon, chopped

Directions:

1. Heat a pan with half of the butter over medium–high heat, add chicken thighs, season with salt, pepper, garlic powder, and onion powder, cook for 3 minutes on each side and transfer to a bowl.

2. Heat the same pan with remaining butter over medium–high heat, add mushrooms, stir, and cook for 5 minutes.

3. Add mustard and water and stir well. Return chicken pieces to pan, stir, cover, and cook for 15 minutes.

4. Add the tarragon, stir, cook for 5 minutes, divide on plates, and serve.

Nutrition:

- Calories 204

- Fat 6.5g

- Carbs 27.9g

- Protein 10.4g

- Sugars 6.9g

Chicken with Olive Tapenade

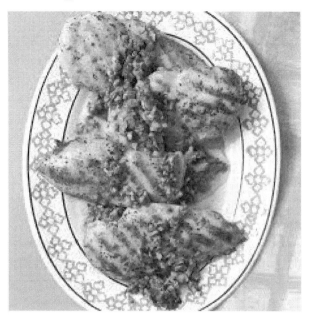

Preparation Time: 10 minutes

Cooking time: 10 minutes

Servings: 6

Ingredients:

- 1 chicken breast, cut into 4 pieces

- 2 tablespoons coconut oil

- 3 garlic cloves, peeled, and crushed

- ½ cup olive tapenade

- For the tapenade:

- 1 cup black olives, pitted

- Salt and ground black pepper, to taste

- 2 tablespoons olive oil

- ¼ cup fresh parsley, chopped

- 1 tablespoons lemon juice

Directions:

1. In a food processor, mix olives with salt, pepper, 2 tablespoons olive oil, lemon juice, and parsley, blend well, and transfer to a bowl.

2. Heat a pan with coconut oil over medium heat, add garlic, stir, and cook for 2 minutes.

3. Add chicken pieces and cook for 4 minutes on each side.

4. Divide chicken on plates and top with the olive's tapenade.

Nutrition:

- Calories 92

- Fat 5.4g

- Carbs 8.1g

- Protein 3.8g

- Sugars 5.1g

Creamy Chicken Casserole

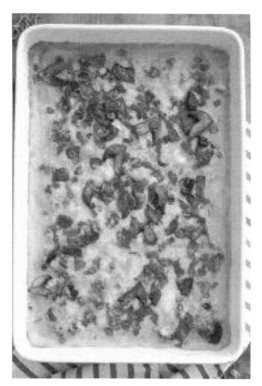

Preparation and Cooking Time: 45 minutes

Servings: 6

Ingredients:

- 2 lbs. chicken thighs

- 2 tablespoon green pesto

- ⅔ lb. cauliflower

- 4 oz. cherry tomatoes

- 7 oz. shredded cheese

- 3 tablespoon butter

- 1¼ cups heavy whipping cream

- 1 leek

- ½ tablespoon lemon juice

- salt and pepper

Directions:

1. Preheat oven to 400 □F.

2. Mix the cream with pesto and lemon juice. Add salt and pepper to taste.

3. Season the chicken with salt and pepper.

4. Fry the chicken thighs in butter until lightly golden.

5. Place the chicken in a baking dish and pour the cream mixture on top.

6. Top the chicken with this mixture.

7. Sprinkle cheese on top and bake for 30 minutes.

Nutrition:

- Calories 125

- Fat 9.4g

- Carbs 8.1g

- Protein 4.2g

- Sugars 1.8g

Garlic Chicken

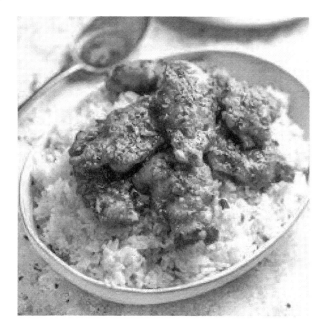

Preparation and Cooking Time: 60 minutes

Servings: 6

Ingredients:

- 8 tablespoons of finely chopped fresh parsley

- 2½ lbs. chicken thighs

- 5 – 10 sliced garlic cloves

- 1 tablespoon of lemon juice

- 2 tablespoon of olive oil

- 4 tablespoons of butter

- Salt and pepper

Directions:

1. Preheat oven to 400 ☐F.

2. Grease a baking pan with butter and place the chicken thighs on it.

3. Sprinkle salt and pepper as desired.

4. Sprinkle garlic and parsley over the chicken pieces.

5. Drizzle lemon juice and olive oil on top.

6. Bake until chicken is golden in color, and the garlic is lightly toasted.

Nutrition:

- Calories 355
- Fat 16.7g
- Carbs 47.7g
- Protein 8.4g
- Sugars 5.8g

Pan–seared Duck Breast

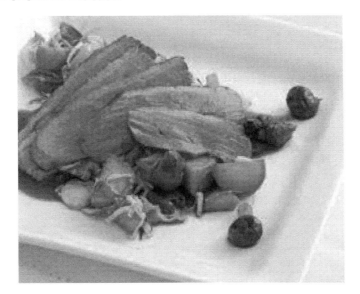

Preparation Time: 10 minutes

Cooking time: 20 minutes

Servings: 6

Ingredients:

- 1 medium duck breast, skin scored

- 1 tablespoon swerve

- 1 tablespoon heavy cream

- 2 tablespoons butter

- ½ teaspoon orange zest

- Salt and ground black pepper, to taste

- 1 cup baby spinach

- ¼ teaspoon fresh sage

Directions:

1. Heat a pan with butter over medium heat. Once it melts, add swerve and stir until butter browns.

2. Add orange zest and sage, stir, and cook for 2 minutes. Add heavy cream and stir again.

3. Heat another pan over medium–high heat, add duck breast, skin side down, cook for 4 minutes, flip, and cook for another 3 minutes.

4. Pour orange sauce over duck breast, stir, and cook for a few minutes.

5. Add spinach to pan with the sauce, stir, and cook for 1 minute.

6. Take duck off heat, slice duck breast, and arrange on a plate.

7. Drizzle orange sauce on top and serve with the spinach on the side.

Nutrition:

- Calories 186
- Fat 7.7g
- Carbs 22.8g
- Protein 7.6g
- Sugars 4g

Duck Breast with Vegetables

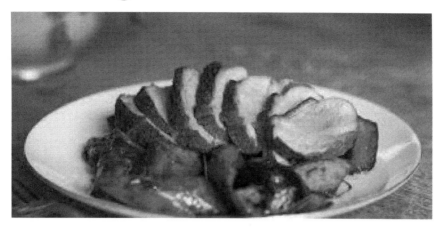

Preparation Time: 10 minutes

Cooking time: 10 minutes

Servings: 6

Ingredients:

- 2 duck breasts, skin on and sliced thin
- 2 zucchinis, sliced
- 1 tablespoon coconut oil
- 1 green onion bunch, chopped
- 1 daikon, chopped
- 2 green bell peppers, seeded and chopped
- Salt and ground black pepper, to taste

Directions:

1. Heat a pan with oil over medium–high heat, add green onions, stir, and cook for 2 minutes.

2. Add zucchini, daikon, bell peppers, salt, pepper, stir, and cook for 10 minutes.

3. Heat another pan over medium–high heat, add duck slices, cook for 3 minutes on each side, and transfer to pan with vegetables. Cook for 3 minutes, divide on plates, and serve.

Nutrition: 184 Calories - 7.2g Fat - 27.1g Carbs - 4.8g Protein - 17.8g Sugars

Duck Breast Salad

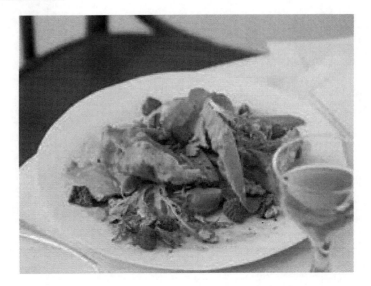

Preparation Time: 10 minutes

Cooking time: 15 minutes

Servings: 6

Ingredients:

- 1 tablespoon swerve

- 1 shallot, peeled and chopped

- ¼ cup red vinegar

- ¼ cup olive oil

- ¼ cup water

- ¾ cup raspberries

- 1 tablespoon Dijon mustard

- Salt and ground black pepper, to taste

- For the salad:

- 10 ounces baby spinach

- 2 medium duck breasts, boneless

- 4 ounces goats' cheese, crumbled

- Salt and ground black pepper, to taste

- ½ pint raspberries

- ½ cup pecans halves

Directions:

1. In a blender, mix the swerve with shallot, vinegar, water, oil, ¾ cup raspberries, mustard, salt, pepper, and blend well.

2. Strain into a bowl and leave aside.

3. Score duck breast, season with salt, pepper, and place skin side down into a pan heated over medium–high heat.

4. Cook for 8 minutes, flip, and cook for 5 minutes.

5. Divide spinach on plates, sprinkle the goat's cheese, pecan halves, and ½ pint raspberries.

6. Slice duck breasts and add on top of raspberries.

7. Drizzle raspberries vinaigrette on top and serve.

Nutrition:

- Calories 218

- Fat 16.9g

- Carbs 15.6g

- Protein 4.4g

- Sugars 0.5g

Turkey Pie

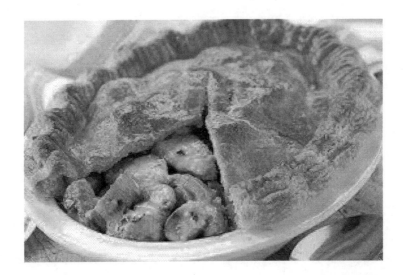

Preparation Time: 10 minutes

Cooking time: 40 minutes

Servings: 6

Ingredients:

- 2 cups turkey stock
- 1 cup turkey meat, cooked and shredded
- Salt and ground black pepper, to taste
- 1 teaspoon fresh thyme, chopped
- ½ cup kale, chopped
- ½ cup butternut squash, peeled and chopped
- ½ cup cheddar cheese, shredded
- ¼ teaspoon paprika
- ¼ teaspoon garlic powder
- ¼ teaspoon xanthan gum
- Vegetable oil cooking spray
- For the crust:

- ¼ cup butter

- ¼ teaspoon xanthan gum

- 2 cups almond flour

- A pinch of salt

- 1 egg

- ¼ cup cheddar cheese

Directions:

1. Heat a saucepan with the stock over medium heat. Add squash and turkey meat, stir, and cook for 10 minutes.

2. Add garlic powder, kale, thyme, paprika, salt, pepper, ½ cup cheddar cheese, and stir well. In a bowl, mix ¼ teaspoon xanthan gum with ½ cup stock from the pan, stir well, and add everything to the saucepan.

3. Take off heat and set aside. In a bowl, mix flour with ¼ teaspoon xanthan gum and a pinch of salt and stir.

4. Add butter, egg, ¼ cup cheddar cheese, and stir until a pie crust dough form. Shape into a ball and place in refrigerator.

5. Spray a baking dish with cooking spray and spread pie filling on the bottom. Transfer dough to a working surface, roll into a circle, and top filling.

6. Press well, and seal edges, place in an oven at 350°F, and bake for 35 minutes.

7. Let the pie to cool and serve.

Nutrition:

- Calories 92

- Fat 5.6 g

- Carbohydrates 10.8 g

- Sugar 2.9 g

- Protein 2.8 g

- Cholesterol 0 mg

Turkey Soup

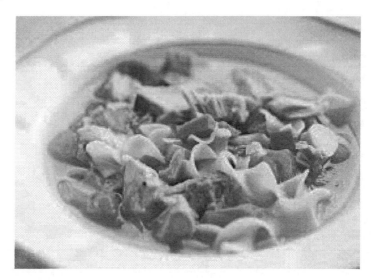

Preparation Time: 10 minutes

Cooking time: 30 minutes

Servings: 6

Ingredients:

- 3 celery stalks, chopped

- 1 onion, peeled and chopped

- 1 tablespoon butter

- 6 cups turkey stock

- Salt and ground black pepper, to taste

- ¼ cup fresh parsley, chopped

- 3 cups baked spaghetti squash, chopped

- 3 cups turkey, cooked, and shredded

Directions:

1. Heat a pot with butter over medium–high heat, add celery and onion, stir, and cook for 5 minutes.

2. Add parsley, stock, turkey meat, salt, and pepper, stir, and cook for 20 minutes.

3. Add spaghetti squash, stir, and cook turkey soup for 10 minutes. Divide into bowls and serve.

Nutrition:

- Calories 189

- Fat 7.5 g

- Carbohydrates 29.2 g

- Sugar 3.3 g

- Protein 3.4 g

- Cholesterol 0 mg

SEAFOOD

Red Cabbage Tilapia Taco Bowl

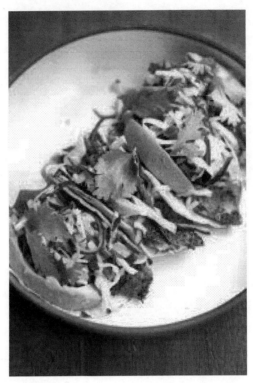

Preparation Time: 10 minutes

Cooking time: 15 minutes

Servings: 6

Ingredients

- 2 cups cauli rice

- 2 tsp ghee

- 4 tilapia fillets, cut into cubes

- ¼ tsp taco seasoning

- Salt and chili pepper to taste

- ¼ head red cabbage, shredded

- 1 ripe avocado, pitted and chopped

Directions

1. Sprinkle cauli rice in a bowl with a little water and microwave for 3 minutes. Fluff after with a fork and set aside.

2. Melt ghee in a skillet over medium heat, rub the tilapia with the taco seasoning, salt, and chili pepper, and fry until brown on all sides, for about 8 minutes in total.

3. Transfer to a plate and set aside. In 4 serving bowls, share the cauli rice, cabbage, fish, and avocado. Serve with chipotle lime sour cream dressing.

Nutrition:

- Calories 441
- Total Fat: 12.7g
- Carbs: 71.5g
- Sugars: 2.7g
- Protein: 10.4g

Sicilian-Style Zoodle Spaghetti

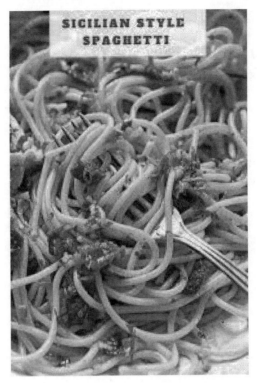

Preparation Time: 10 minutes

Cooking time: 15 minutes

Servings: 6

Ingredients

- 4 cups zoodles (spiralled zucchini)

- 2 ounces cubed bacon

- 4 ounces canned sardines, ch opped

- ½ cup canned chopped tomatoes

- 1 tbsp capers

- 1 tbsp parsley

- 1 tsp minced garlic

Directions

1. Pour some of the sardine oil in a pan.

2. Add garlic and cook for 1 minute.

3. Add the bacon and cook for 2 more minutes. Stir in the tomatoes and let simmer for 5 minutes.

4. Add zoodles and sardines and cook for 3 minutes.

Baked Nutty Halibut

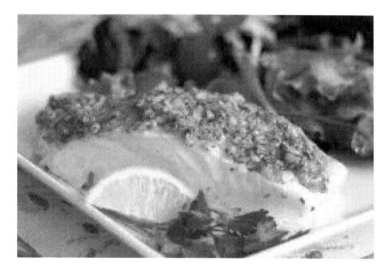

Preparation Time: 20 minutes

Cooking Time: 15 minutes

Servings: 4

Ingredients:

- ½ cup heavy (whipping) cream

- ½ cup finely chopped pecans

- ¼ cup finely chopped almonds

- 4 (4-ounce) boneless halibut fillets

- Sea salt

- Freshly ground black pepper

- 2 tablespoons extra-virgin olive oil

Directions:

1. Preheat the oven to 400°F. Line a baking sheet with parchment.

2. Pour the heavy cream into a bowl and set it on your work surface.

3. In another bowl, stir together the pecans and almonds and set beside the cream.

4. Pat the halibut fillets dry with paper towels and lightly season with salt and pepper.

5. Dip the fillets in the cream, shaking off the excess; then dredge the fish in the nut mixture so that both sides of each piece are thickly coated.

6. Place the fish on the prepared baking sheet and brush both sides of the pieces generously with olive oil.

7. Bake the fish until the topping is golden and the fish flakes easily with a fork, 12 to 15 minutes. Serve.

8. Make Ahead: The "breaded" fish fillets can be completely put together and then frozen on a baking sheet. Transfer the individual fillets to plastic bags and freeze for up to 1 month. Cook the fillets from frozen, brushed lightly with olive oil, in a 350°F oven for about 35 minutes.

Nutrition:

- Calories 212

- Total Fat: 6.6g

- Carbs: 34.9g

- Sugars: 12.2g

- Protein: 8.9g

Sour Cream Salmon with Parmesan

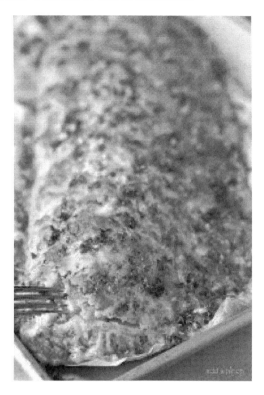

Preparation Time: 10 minutes

Cooking time: 20 minutes

Servings: 6

Ingredients

- 1 cup sour cream
- ½ tbsp minced dill
- ½ lemon, zested and juiced
- Pink salt and black pepper to season
- 4 salmon steaks
- ½ cup grated Parmesan cheese

Directions

1. Preheat oven to 400°F and line a baking sheet with parchment paper; set aside. In a bowl, mix the sour cream, dill, lemon zest, juice, salt, and black pepper, and set aside.

2. Season the fish with salt and black pepper, drizzle lemon juice on both sides of the fish and arrange them in the baking sheet. Spread the sour cream mixture on each fish and sprinkle with Parmesan.

3. Bake the fish for 15 minutes and after broil the top for 2 minutes with a close watch for a nice a brown color. Plate the fish and serve with buttery green beans.

Nutrition:

- Calories 251

- Fat 6.2g

- Carbs 44.1g

- Protein 4.2g

- Sugars 3g

Sushi Shrimp Rolls

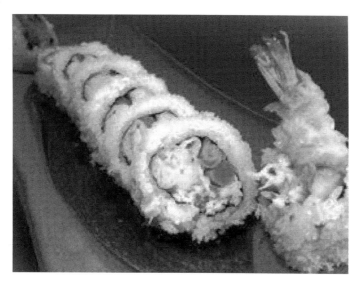

Preparation Time: 10 minutes

Cooking time: 20 minutes

Servings: 6

Ingredients

- 2 cups cooked and chopped shrimp

- 1 tbsp sriracha sauce

- ¼ cucumber, julienned

- 5 hand roll nori sheets

- ¼ cup mayonnaise

Directions

1. Combine shrimp, mayonnaise, cucumber and sriracha sauce in a bowl. Lay out a single nori sheet on a flat surface and spread about 1/5 of the shrimp mixture.

2. Roll the nori sheet as desired.

3. Repeat with the other ingredients. Serve with sugar-free soy sauce.

Nutrition: 233 Calories - 3.3g Fat - 45.8g Carbs - 5.8g Protein - 8.7g Sugars

Grilled Shrimp with Chimichurri Sauce

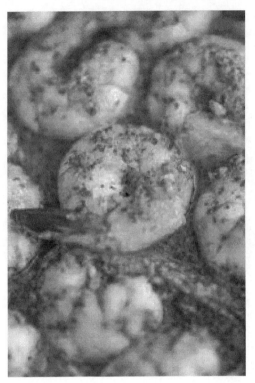

Preparation Time: 10 minutes

Cooking time: 20 minutes

Servings: 6

Ingredients

- 1 pound shrimp, peeled and deveined

- 2 tbsp olive oil

- Juice of 1 lime

- Chimichurri

- ½ tsp salt

- ¼ cup olive oil

- 2 garlic cloves

- ¼ cup red onions, chopped

- ¼ cup red wine vinegar

- ½ tsp pepper

- 2 cups parsley

- ¼ tsp red pepper flakes

Directions

4. Process the chimichurri ingredients in a blender until smooth; set aside.

5. Combine shrimp, olive oil, and lime juice, in a bowl, and let marinate in the fridge for 30 minutes.

6. Preheat your grill to medium. Add shrimp and cook about 2 minutes per side. Serve shrimp drizzled with the chimichurri sauce.

Nutrition:

- Calories 194

- Fat 5.4g

- Carbs 29.9g

- Protein 8g

- Sugars 5.1g

Coconut Crab Patties

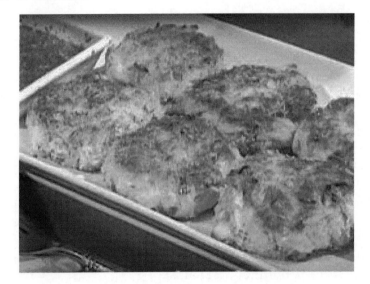

Preparation Time: 10 minutes

Cooking time: 50 minutes

Servings: 6

Ingredients

- 2 tbsp coconut oil
- 1 tbsp lemon juice
- 1 cup lump crab meat
- 2 tsp Dijon mustard
- 1 egg, beaten
- 1 ½ tbsp coconut flour

Directions

1. In a bowl to the crabmeat, add all the ingredients, except for the oil; mix well to combine.

2. Make patties out of the mixture. Melt the coconut oil in a skillet over medium heat. Add the crab patties and cook for about 2-3 minutes per side.

Nutrition: Calories 277 - Fat 26.2g - Carbs 9g - Sugar 4g - Protein 7.5g – Cholesterol 31mg

Shrimp in Curry Sauce

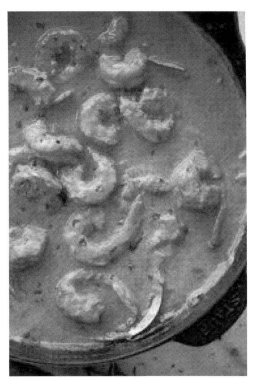

Preparation Time: 10 minutes

Cooking time: 20 minutes

Servings: 6

Ingredients

- ½ ounce grated Parmesan cheese

- 1 egg, beaten

- ¼ tsp curry powder

- 2 tsp almond flour

- 12 shrimp, shelled

- 3 tbsp coconut oil

- Sauce

- 2 tbsp curry leaves

- 2 tbsp butter

- ½ onion, diced

- ½ cup heavy cream

- ½ ounce cheddar cheese, shredded

Directions

1. Combine all dry ingredients for the batter.

2. Melt the coconut oil in a skillet over medium heat. Dip the shrimp in the egg first, and then coat with the dry mixture. Fry until golden and crispy.

3. In another skillet, melt butter.

4. Add onion and cook for 3 minutes.

5. Add curry leaves and cook for 30 seconds. Stir in heavy cream and cheddar and cook until thickened.

6. Add shrimp and coat well.

7. Serve.

Nutrition:

- Calories 190

- Fat 16.3 g

- Carbohydrates 2.3 g

- Sugar 0.2 g

- Protein 8.7 g

- Cholesterol 52 mg

Tilapia with Olives & Tomato Sauce

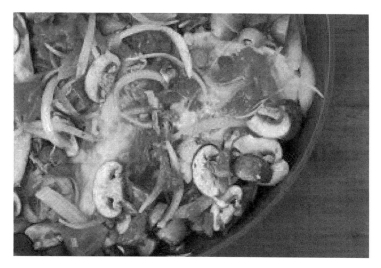

Preparation Time: 10 minutes

Cooking time: 50 minutes

Servings: 6

Ingredients

- 4 tilapia fillets

- 2 garlic cloves, minced

- 2 tsp oregano

- 14 ounces diced tomatoes

- 1 tbsp olive oil

- ½ red onion, chopped

- 2 tbsp parsley

- ¼ cup kalamata olives

Directions

1. Heat olive oil in a skillet over medium heat and cook the onion for 3 minutes.

2. Add garlic and oregano and cook for 30 seconds. Stir in tomatoes and bring the mixture to a boil. Reduce the heat and simmer for 5 minutes.

3. Add olives and tilapia and cook for about 8 minutes.

4. Serve the tilapia with tomato sauce.

Nutrition:

- Calories 66
- Fat 3.3 g
- Carbohydrates 9.9 g
- Sugar 5.1 g
- Protein 0.8 g
- Cholesterol 9 mg

Lemon Garlic Shrimp

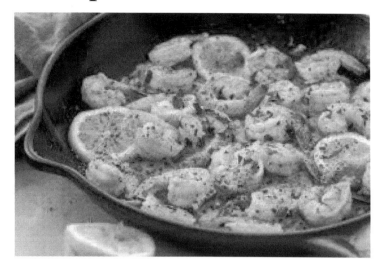

Preparation Time: 10 minutes

Cooking time: 50 minutes

Servings: 6

Ingredients

- ½ cup butter, divided

- 2 lb. shrimp, peeled and deveined

- Salt and black pepper to taste

- ¼ tsp sweet paprika

- 1 tbsp minced garlic

- 3 tbsp water

- 1 lemon, zested and juiced

- 2 tbsp chopped parsley

Directions

1. Melt half of the butter in a large skillet over medium heat, season the shrimp with salt, black pepper, paprika, and add to the butter.

2. Stir in the garlic and cook the shrimp for 4 minutes on both sides until pink. Remove to a bowl and set aside.

3. Put the remaining butter in the skillet; include the lemon zest, juice, and water.

4. Add the shrimp, parsley, and adjust the taste with salt and pepper.

5. Cook for 2 minutes.

6. Serve shrimp and sauce with squash pasta.

Nutrition:

- Calories 245

- Fat 7.5 g

- Carbohydrates 32.8 g

- Sugar 3.5 g

- Protein 11.8 g

- Cholesterol 22 mg

Seared Scallops with Chorizo and Asiago Cheese

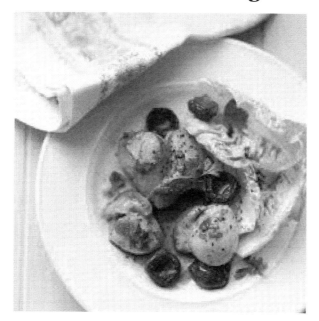

Preparation Time: 10 minutes

Cooking time: 30 minutes

Servings: 6

Ingredients

- 2 tbsp ghee

- 16 fresh scallops

- 8 ounces chorizo, chopped

- 1 red bell pepper, seeds removed, sliced

- 1 cup red onions, finely chopped

- 1 cup asiago cheese, grated

- Salt and black pepper to taste

Directions

1. Melt half of the ghee in a skillet over medium heat and cook the onion and bell pepper for 5 minutes until tender.

2. Add the chorizo and stir-fry for another 3 minutes. Remove and set aside.

3. Pat dry the scallops with paper towels, and season with salt and pepper.

4. Add the remaining ghee to the skillet and sear the scallops for 2 minutes on each side to have a golden-brown color.

5. Add the chorizo mixture back and warm through. Transfer to serving platter and top with asiago cheese.

Nutrition:

- Calories 78

- Fat 4.9 g

- Carbohydrates 8.5 g

- Sugar 4.4 g

- Protein 2 g

- Cholesterol 0 mg

Tuna Cakes

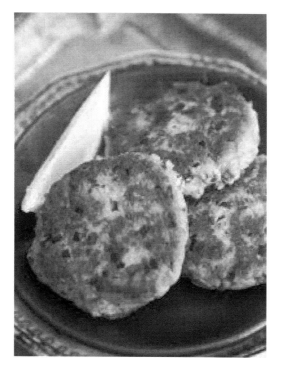

Preparation Time: 10 minutes

Cooking time: 10 minutes

Servings: 12

Ingredients:

- 15 ounces canned tuna, drained well and flaked

- 2 eggs

- ½ teaspoon dried dill

- 1 teaspoon dried parsley

- ½ cup onion chopped

- 1 teaspoon garlic powder

- Salt and ground black pepper, to taste

- Oil, for frying

Directions:

1. In a bowl, mix tuna with salt, pepper, dill, parsley, onion, garlic powder, eggs, and stir well.

2. Shape tuna cakes and place on a plate.

3. Heat a pan with oil over medium–high heat, add tuna cakes, cook for 5 minutes on each side. Divide on plates and serve.

Nutrition:

- Calories 322
- Fat 7.8 g
- Carbohydrates 44.3 g
- Sugar 7.3 g
- Protein 20.7 g
- Cholesterol 13 mg

Pan–roasted Cod

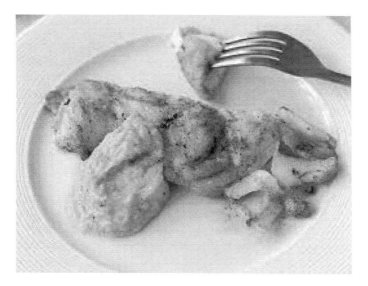

Preparation Time: 10 minutes

Cooking time: 20 minutes

Servings: 4

Ingredients:

- 1-pound cod, cut into medium–sized pieces

- Salt and ground black pepper, to t aste

- 2 green onions, chopped

- 2 garlic cloves, peeled and minced

- 2 tablespoons soy sauce

- 1 cup fish stock

- 1 tablespoon balsamic vinegar

- 1 tablespoon fresh ginger, grated

- ½ teaspoon red chili flakes

Directions:

1. Heat a pan over medium–high heat, add fish pieces, and brown on each side.

2. Add garlic, green onions, salt, pepper, soy sauce, fish stock, vinegar, chili pepper, ginger, stir, cover, reduce heat, and cook for 20 minutes.

3. Divide on plates and serve.

Nutrition:

- Calories 142

- Fat 5.9 g

- Carbohydrates 17 g

- Sugar 2.2 g

- Protein 6.3 g

- Cholesterol 0 mg

Sea Bass with Capers

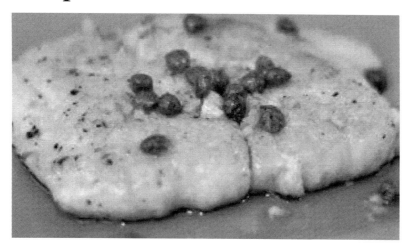

Preparation Time: 10 minutes

Cooking time: 15 minutes

Servings: 4

Ingredients:

- 1 lemon, sliced

- 1-pound sea bass fillet

- 2 tablespoons capers

- 2 tablespoons fresh dill

- Salt and ground black pepper, to taste

Directions:

1. Put sea bass fillet into a baking dish, season with salt, and pepper, add capers, dill, and lemon slices on top.

2. Place in an oven at 350°F and bake for 15 minutes.

Nutrition:

- Calories 55

- Fat 0.4 g

- Carbohydrates 11.6 g

- Sugar 5 g

- Protein 3.4 g

- Cholesterol 0 mg

Cod with Arugula

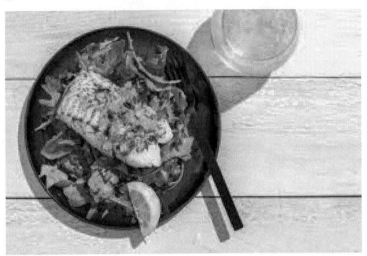

Preparation Time: 10 minutes

Cooking time: 20 minutes

Servings: 4

Ingredients:

- 2 cod fillets

- 1 tablespoon olive oil

- Salt and ground black pepper, to taste

- Juice of 1 lemon

- cup arugula

- ½ cup black olives, pitted and sliced

- 2 tablespoons capers

- 1 garlic clove, peeled and chopped

Directions:

1. Arrange fish fillets in a heatproof dish, season with salt, pepper, drizzle the oil and lemon juice, toss to coat, place in an oven at 450°F, and bake for 20 minutes.

2. In a food processor, mix arugula with salt, pepper, capers, olives, garlic, and blend well.

3. Arrange the fish on plates, top with arugula tapenade, and serve.

Nutrition:

- Calories 240
- Total Fats 12g
- Carbs: 12g
- Protein 28g
- Dietary Fiber: 2.5g

Baked Halibut with Vegetables

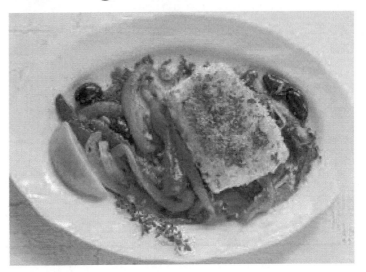

Preparation Time: 10 minutes

Cooking time: 35 minutes

Servings: 4

Ingredients:

- 1 red bell pepper, seeded and chopped

- 1 yellow bell pepper, seeded and chopped

- 1 teaspoon balsamic vinegar

- 1 tablespoon olive oil

- 2 halibut fillets

- 2 cups baby spinach

- Salt and ground black pepper, to taste

- 1 teaspoon cumin

Directions:

1. In a bowl, mix bell peppers with salt, pepper, half of the oil, and vinegar, toss to coat well, and transfer to a baking dish.

2. Place in oven at 400°F and bake for 20 minutes.

3. Heat a pan with the rest of the oil over medium heat, add fish, season with salt, pepper, cumin, and brown on all sides.

4. Take baking dish out of the oven, add the spinach, stir gently, and divide the whole mixture on plates.

5. Add fish on the side, sprinkle with salt and pepper, and serve.

Nutrition:

- Calories 240
- Total Fats 0.2g
- Carbs: 9g
- Protein 20g
- Dietary Fiber: 2g

Fish Curry

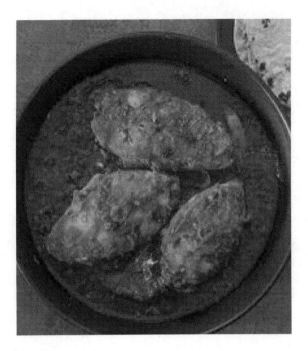

Preparation Time: 10 minutes

Cooking time: 25 minutes

Servings: 4

Ingredients:

- 4 white fish fillets

- ½ teaspoon mustard seeds

- Salt and ground black pepper, to taste

- 2 green chilies, chopped

- 1 teaspoon fresh ginger, grated

- 1 teaspoon curry powder

- ¼ teaspoon cumin

- tablespoons coconut oil

- 1 onion, peeled and chopped

- 1–inch turmeric root, grated

- ¼ cup fresh cilantro

- 1½ cups coconut cream

- garlic cloves, peeled and minced

Directions:

1. Heat a saucepan with half of the coconut oil over medium heat, add mustard seeds, and cook for 2 minutes.

2. Add ginger, onion, garlic, stir, and cook for 5 minutes. Add turmeric, curry powder, chilies, and cumin, stir, and cook for 5 minutes.

3. Add coconut milk, salt, and pepper, stir, bring to a boil, and cook for 15 minutes.

4. Heat another pan with remaining oil over medium heat, add fish, stir, and cook for 3 minutes.

5. Add to curry sauce, stir, and cook for 5 minutes.

6. Add cilantro, stir, divide into bowls, and serve.

Nutrition:

- Calories 240

- Total Fats 0.2g

- Carbs: 9g

- Protein 20g

- Dietary Fiber: 2g

Keto Baked Tilapia with Cherry Tomatoes

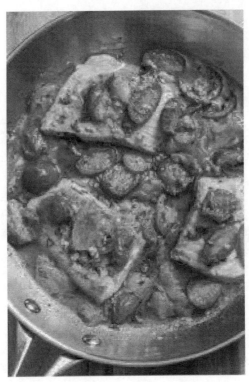

Preparation Time: 10 minutes

Cooking time: 25 minutes

Servings: 4

Ingredients Needed:

- Butter (2 tsp.)

- Tilapia fillets (2 - 4 oz. each)

- Cherry tomatoes (8)

- Pitted black olives (.25 cup)

- Salt (.5 tsp.)

- Paprika (.25 tsp.)

- Black pepper (.25 tsp.)

- Garlic powder (1 tsp.)

- Lemon juice (1 tbsp.)

- Optional: Balsamic vinegar (1 tbsp.)

Directions

1. Warm the oven to reach 375° F.

2. Grease a roasting pan and add the butter along with the olives and tomatoes.

3. Season the tilapia with the spices. Squeeze the lemon and spritz the fish fillets, adding them to the pan.

4. Add a piece of foil over the pan. Bake until the fish easily flakes (25 to 30 min.).

5. Garnish with the vinegar if desired.

Nutrition:

- Calories 84

- Fat 2.1 g

- Carbohydrates 14.7 g

- Sugar 3.2 g

- Protein 3.3 g

- Cholesterol 5 mg

Keto Bun less Burger

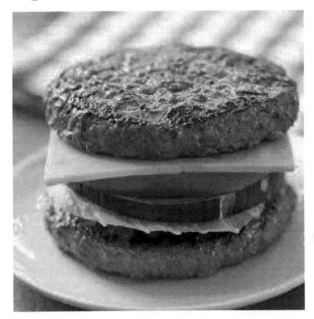

Preparation Time: 10 minutes

Cooking time: 20 minutes

Servings: 4

Ingredients Needed:

- Olive oil/bacon drippings (2 tbsp.)

- Ground beef (1 lb.)

- Worcestershire sauce (1 tbsp.)

- McCormick's Montreal Steak Seasoning (1 tbsp.)

- Sliced onions (4 oz.)

Directions

1. Warm the grill. Clean and oil the grate.

2. Combine the beef, salt, pepper, olive oil, Worcestershire sauce, and seasonings.

3. Grill the burger until you reach the desired degree of doneness.

4. Enjoy with your favorite side dishes.

5. Prepare the onions by adding one tablespoon of oil in a skillet using the med-low heat setting. When heated, add the onion and sauté until softened.

Nutrition:

- Calories: 215

- Carbohydrates: 20.7g

- Protein:7.3 g

- Fat: 12.2g

- Sugar: 10.2g

- Sodium: 1335mg

Keto Chuck Steak - Slow-Cooked

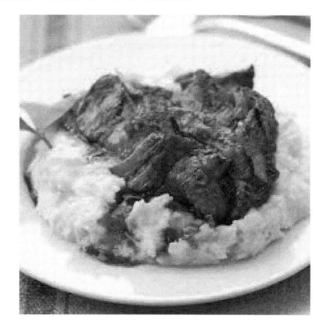

Preparation Time: 10 minutes

Cooking time: 20 minutes

Servings: 4

Ingredients Needed:

- Chuck steak (4.5 lb.)

- Celery stalks (4)

- Carrots (3)

- Garlic cloves (2)

- Beef stock (2 cups)

- Red wine (1 cup)

- Pepper and salt (to your liking)

Directions

1. Pour 1 inch of water into the cooker. Add the roast and prepare using the high setting for four hours. Slice the veggies and toss them around the roast.

2. Empty the wine and broth over the meat and add all the spices.

3. Simmer for four more hours on the high setting.

4. Slice the steak into eight servings and serve with the veggies.

Nutrition:

- Calories: 229

- Carbohydrates:7.3g

- Protein: 12.1 g

- Fat: 17.5g

- Sugar: 4.1g

- Sodium: 555mg

Keto Crockpot Spaghetti & Pesto Meatballs

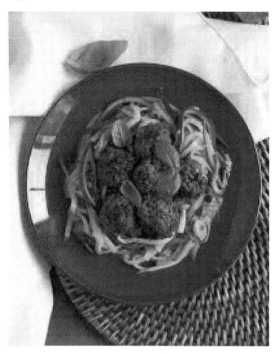

Preparation Time: 10 minutes

Cooking time: 35 minutes

Servings: 4

Ingredients Needed:

- The Meatballs:
- Ground beef - 90% lean (1 lb.)
- Olive oil (1 tbsp.)
- Beef broth (2 cups)

The Pesto:

- Basil leaves (1.5 cups)
- Olive oil (.33 cup + more as needed)
- Garlic cloves (2)
- Walnuts/Pine nuts (2 tbsp.)

- Lemon zest & juice (1 lemon)

- Pepper and salt (1 dash each)

The Spaghetti:

- Zucchini (2)

Directions

1. Make the pesto. Blend all the pesto fixings in a mixing bowl. Set aside half of the mixture for serving.

2. Combine the ground beef and the other half of the basil pesto. Shape it into small balls.

3. Warm the olive oil. Add the meatballs using one or two batches, and fry until browned. Add them and the broth to the crockpot.

4. Place a lid on the cooker and set the timer for two hours, spooning the broth over the meatballs frequently.

5. Spiralize and add the zucchini noodles in with the rest of the pesto.

6. Serve with a portion of the meatballs on top and a sprinkle of salt and fresh pepper

Nutrition:

- Calories: 191

- Carbohydrates: 21.2g

- Protein: 8.3g

- Fat: 9.1g

- Sugar: 8.8g

- Sodium: 1161mg

Keto Jamaican Jerk Pork Roast

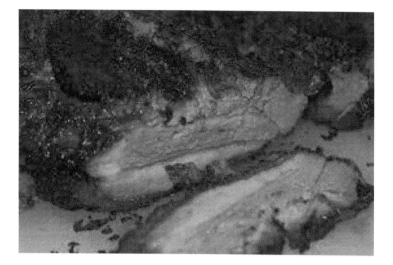

Preparation Time: 10 minutes

Cooking time: 35 minutes

Servings: 4

Ingredients Needed:

- Jamaican Jerk spice blend (.25 cup)

- Olive oil (1 tbsp.)

- Pork shoulder (4 lb.)

- Broth or beef stock (.5 cup)

- Also Needed: Dutch or regular oven

Directions

1. Rub the roast well the oil and coat with the jerk spice blend.

2. Use the Dutch oven to sear the roast on all sides. Add the beef broth.

3. Cover the pot and simmer for about four hours using the low-temperature setting. (You can also bake it for 3 hours at 375° F.).

4. Shred the meat and serve.

Nutrition: Calories 510 - Total Fats 16g - Carbs: 6g - Protein 52g - Dietary Fiber: 1.5g

Keto Spring Seafood & Meat

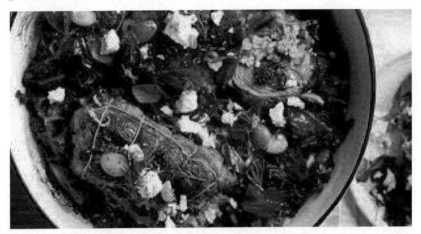

Preparation Time: 10 minutes

Cooking time: 45 minutes

Servings: 4

Ingredients Needed:

- Large eggs (3)

- Smoked salmon (1.8 oz.)

- Avocado (half of 1 average-size)

- Spring onion (1)

- Cream cheese - full-fat (2 tbsp)

- Chives - freshly chopped (2 tbsp.)

- Butter or ghee (1 tbsp.)

- Pepper and salt (as desired)

Directions

1. Add a sprinkle of pepper and salt to the eggs. Use a fork or whisk—mixing them well. Blend in the chives and cream cheese.

2. Prepare the salmon and avocado (peel and slice or chop).

3. Combine the butter/ghee and the egg mixture in a frying pan. Continue cooking on low heat until done.

4. Place the omelet on a serving dish with a portion of cheese over it. Sprinkle the onion, prepared avocado, and salmon into the wrap.

5. Close and serve!

Nutrition:

- Calories 443
- Total Fats 18.4g
- Carbs: 9.7g
- Protein 58.8g
- Dietary Fiber: 1.8g

SMOOTHIES

Green Coconut Smoothie

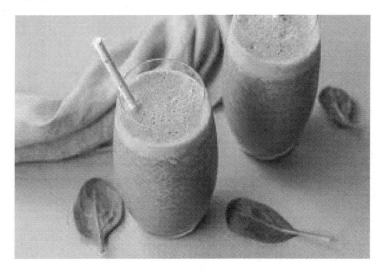

Preparation Time: 10 minutes

Servings: 3

Ingredients:

- 1 1/4 cup coconut milk canned

- 2 Tablespoon chia seeds

- 1 cup of fresh kale leaves

- 1 cup of spinach leaves

- 1 scoop vanilla protein powder

- 1 cup of ice cubes

- Granulated stevia sweetener to taste; optional

- 1/2 cup water

Directions:

1. Rinse and clean kale and the spinach leaves from any dirt.

2. Add all ingredients in your blender.

3. Blend until you get a nice smoothie.

4. Serve into chilled glass.

Nutrition:

- Calories 323
- Total Fats 9.6g
- Carbs: 59.7g
- Protein 9.2g
- Dietary Fiber: 10.6g

Instant Coffee Smoothie

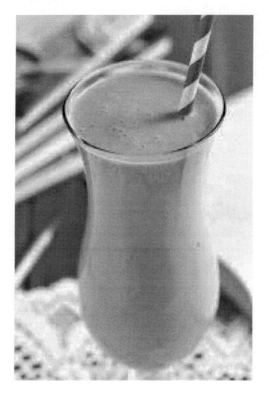

Preparation Time: 20 minutes

Servings: 3

Ingredients:

- 2 cups of instant coffee

- 1 cup almond milk or coconut milk

- 1/4 cup heavy cream

- 2 Tablespoon cocoa powder unsweetened

- 1 - 2 Handful of fresh spinach leaves

- 10 drops liquid stevia

Directions:

1. Make a coffee; set aside.

2. Place all remaining ingredients in your fast-speed blender; blend for 45 - 60 seconds or until done.

3. Pour your instant coffee in a blender and continue to blend for further 30 - 45 seconds.

4. Serve immediately.

Nutrition:

- Calories 338

- Total Fats 29.2g

- Carbs: 18.1g

- Protein 8.8g

- Dietary Fiber: 5.8g

Keto Blood Sugar Adjuster Smoothie

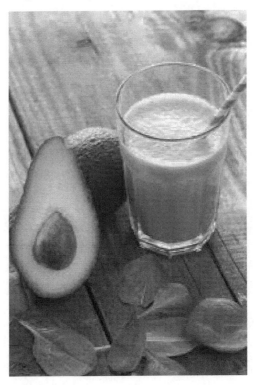

Preparation Time: 10 minutes

Servings: 3

Ingredients:

- 2 cups of green cabbage
- 1/2 avocado
- 1 Tablespoon Apple cider vinegar
- Juice of 1 lemon
- 1 cup of water
- 1 cup of crushed ice cubes for serving

Directions:

1. Place all ingredients in your high-speed blender or in a food processor and blend until smooth and soft. Serve in chilled glasses with crushed ice.

Nutrition: Kcal 243 - Carbs 61g - Fat 1g - Protein 2g

Lime Spinach Smoothie

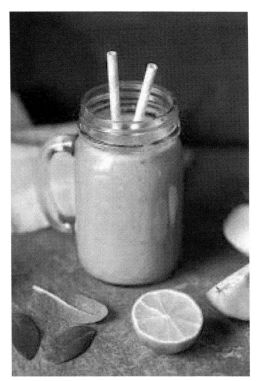

Preparation Time: 5 minutes

Servings: 3

Ingredients:

- 1 cup water

- lime juice 1-2 limes

- 1 green apple cut into chunks; core discarded

- 2 cups fresh spinach, roughly chopped

- 1/2 cup fresh chopped fresh mint

- 1/2 avocado

- Ice crushed

- 1/4 teaspoon ground cinnamon

- 1 Tablespoon natural sweetener of your choice optional

Directions:

1. Place all ingredients in your high-speed blender.

2. Blend for 45 - 60 seconds or until your smoothie is smooth and creamy.

3. Serve in a chilled glass.

4. Adjust sweetener to taste.

Nutrition:

- Kcal 202

- Carbs 23g

- Fat 10g

- Protein 9g

Protein Coconut Smoothie

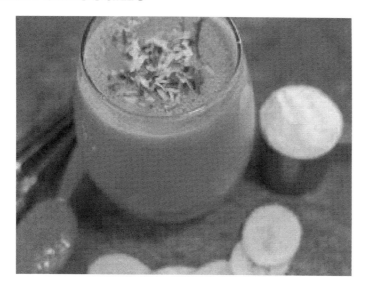

Preparation Time: 15 minutes

Servings: 3

Ingredients:

- 1 1/2 cup of coconut milk canned

- 1 cup of fresh spinach finely chopped

- 1 scoop vanilla protein powder

- 2 Tablespoon chia seeds

- 1 cup of ice cubes crushed

- 2 - 3 Tablespoon Stevia granulated natural sweetener optional

Directions:

1. Rinse and clean your spinach leaves from any dirt.

2. Place all ingredients from the list above in a blender.

3. Blend until you get a smoothie like consistently.

4. Serve into chilled glass and it is ready to drink.

Nutrition: Kcal 287 - Carbs 22g - Fat 14g - Protein 17g

Strong Spinach and Hemp Smoothie

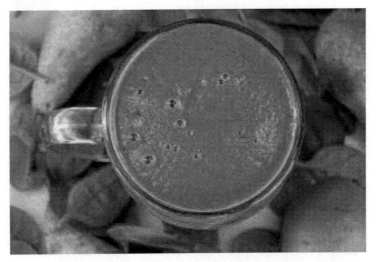

Preparation Time: 10 minutes

Servings: 3

Ingredients:

- 1 cup almond milk
- 1 small ripe banana
- 2 Tablespoon hemp seeds
- 2 handful fresh spinach leaves
- 1 teaspoon pure vanilla extract
- 1 cup of water
- 2 Tablespoon of natural sweetener such Stevia, Truvia…etc.

Directions:

1. First, rinse and clean your spinach leaves from any dirt.
2. Place the spinach in a blender or food processor along with remaining ingredients.
3. Blend for 45 - 60 seconds or until done.
4. Add more or less sweetener.
5. Serve.

Nutrition: Kcal 229 - Carbs 20g - Fat 15g - Protein 9g

Green Low Carb Breakfast Smoothie

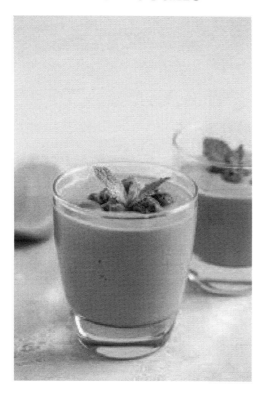

Preparation Time: 5 minutes

Servings: 3

Ingredients:

- 1 oz of spinach

- 2 oz of celery

- 1 ½ cups of almond milk

- 2 oz avocado

- 2 oz of cucumber

- 1 tbsp coconut oil

- 1 scoop of protein powder

- 10 drops of liquid stevia

- ½ tsp of chia seeds

Directions:

1. Add almond milk and spinach to blender.

2. Blend briefly.

3. Add the rest of the ingredients

4. Pour mixture into a glass and sprinkle chia seeds on top.

Nutrition:

- Kcal 276

- Carbs 25g

- Fat 18

- Protein 9g

Total Almond Smoothie

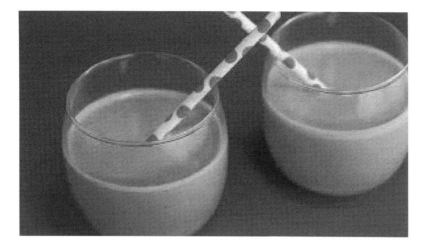

Preparation Time: 15 minutes

Servings: 3

Ingredients:

- 1 1/2 cups of almond milk
- 2 Tablespoon of almond butter
- 2 Tablespoon ground almonds
- 1 cup of fresh kale leaves or to taste
- 1/2 teaspoon of cocoa powder
- 1 Tablespoon chia seeds
- 1/2 cup of water

Directions:

1. Rinse and carefully clean kale leaves from any dirt.
2. Add almond milk, almond butter, and ground almonds in your blender; blend for 45 - 60 seconds.
3. Add kale leaves, cocoa powder, and chia seeds; blend for further 45 seconds.
4. If your smoothie is too thick, pour more almond milk or water.

Nutrition: Kcal 377 - Carbs 37g - Fat 12g - Protein 31g

Ultimate Green Mix Smoothie

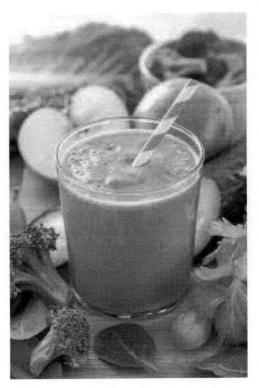

Preparation Time: 15 minutes

Servings: 3

Ingredients:

- Handful of spinach leaves

- Handful of collards greens

- Handful of lettuce, cos or romain

- 1 1/2 cup of almond milk

- 1/2 cup of water

- 1/4 cup of stevia granulated sweetener

- 1 teaspoon pure vanilla extract

- 1 cup crushed ice cubes optional

Directions:

1. Rinse and carefully clean your greens from any dirt.

2. Place all ingredients from the list above in your blender or food processor.

3. Blend until done or 45 - 30 seconds.

4. Serve with or without crushed ice.

Nutrition:

- Kcal 315

- Carbs 17g

- Fat 12g

- Protein 26g

The Strawberry Almond Smoothie

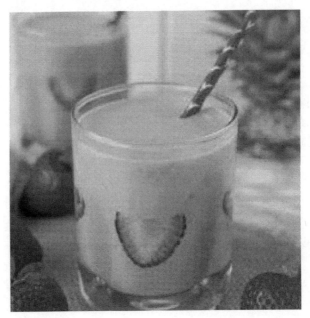

Preparation Time: 10 minutes

Servings: 3

Ingredients:

- 16 ounces unsweetened almond milk, vanilla

- 1 pack stevia

- 4 ounces heavy cream

- 1 scoop vanilla whey protein

- ¼ cup frozen strawberries, unsweetened

Directions:

1. Add all the listed ingredients to a blender.

2. Blend on high until smooth and creamy.

3. Enjoy your smoothie.

Nutrition: Kcal 498 - Carbs 47g - Fat 28g - Protein 26g

Early Morning Fruit Smoothie

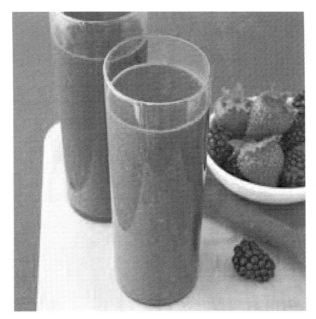

Preparation Time: 10 minutes

Servings: 3

Ingredients:

- 1 cup Spring mix salad blend

- 2 cups water

- 3 medium blackberries, whole

- 1 packet Stevia, optional

- 1 tablespoon avocado oil

- 1 tablespoon coconut flakes shredded and unsweetened

- 2 tablespoons pecans, chopped

- 1 tablespoon hemp seed

- 1 tablespoon sunflower seed

Directions:

1. Add all the listed ingredients to a blender.

2. Blend on high until smooth and creamy.

3. Enjoy your smoothie.

Nutrition:

- Kcal 355

- Carbs 8g

- Fat 12g

- Protein 27g

Banana Chai Smoothie with Cinnamon

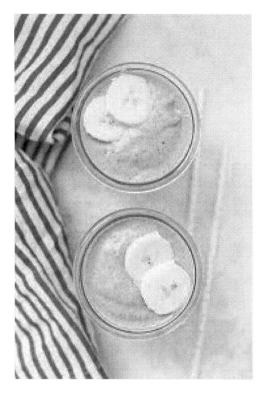

Preparation time: 10 minutes

Servings: 3

Ingredients:

- 1 16-ounce cupful of brewed chai tea, cooled d
- ½ cup unsweetened vanilla almond milk
- 1 teaspoon vanilla extract
- 1 frozen banana
- ½ teaspoon cinnamon
- ice cubes

Directions:

1. Place the tea, almond milk, vanilla, banana, cinnamon, and ice cubes in a blender and process at high speed until smooth and creamy. Pour into glasses and enjoy.

Nutrition: Kcal 288 - Carbs 39g - Fat 13g - Protein 6g

Berry Banana with Quinoa Smoothie

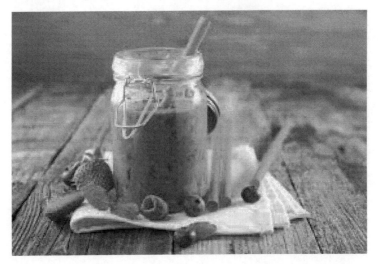

Preparation time: 10 minutes

Servings: 3

Ingredients:

- ½ cup cooked quinoa, chilled
- 1 frozen banana
- 1 cup frozen raspberries or strawberries
- 1½ cups green tea, brewed and cooled
- ice cubes

Directions:

1. Place the quinoa, frozen banana sections, berries, and tea in the blender.
2. Process until smooth. Serve.

Nutrition:

- Calories 146
- Total Fat: 4.5 g
- Carbs: 23.5 g
- Sugars: 16.4 g
- Protein: 5.4 g

SALAD CONDIMENTS, SAUCES, AND SPREADS

Sautéed Celeriac with Tomato Sauce

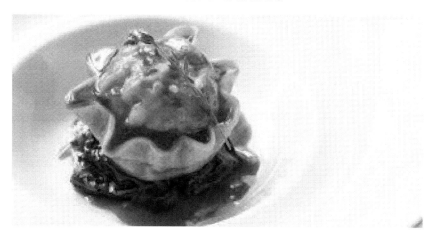

Preparation Time: 10 minutes

Cooking Time: 70 minutes

Servings: 6

Ingredients

- 2 tbsp olive oil
- 1 garlic clove, crushed
- 1 celeriac, sliced
- ¼ cup vegetable stock
- Salt and black pepper, to taste
- For the sauce
- 2 tomatoes, halved
- 2 tbsp olive oil
- ½ cup onions, chopped
- 2 cloves garlic, minced

- 1 chili, minced

- 1 bunch fresh basil, chopped

- 1 tbsp fresh cilantro, chopped

- Salt and black pepper, to taste

Directions

1. Set a pan over medium heat and warm olive oil. Add in garlic and sauté for 1 minute. Stir in celeriac slices, stock, and cook until softened. Sprinkle with black pepper and salt; kill the heat.

2. Brush olive oil to the tomato halves. Microwave for 15 minutes; get rid of any excess liquid.

3. Remove the cooked tomatoes to a food processor; add the rest of the ingredients for the sauce and puree to obtain the desired consistency.

4. Serve the celeriac topped with tomato sauce.

Nutrition:

- Calories 248

- Fat 2.5 g

- Carbohydrates 51.4 g

- Sugar 9.4 g

- Protein 10.6 g

- Cholesterol 0 mg

Cauliflower Mac and Cheese

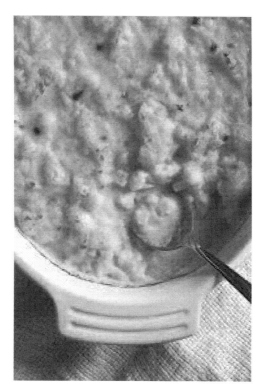

Preparation Time: 10 minutes

Cooking Time:20 minutes

Servings: 6

Ingredients

- 1 cauliflower head, riced

- 1 ½ cups shredded mozzarella cheese

- 2 tsp paprika

- ¾ tsp rosemary

- 2 tsp turmeric

- Salt and black pepper to taste

Directions

1. Microwave the cauliflower for 5 minutes.

2. Place it in cheesecloth and squeeze the extra juices out. Place the cauli in a pot over medium heat.

3. Add paprika, turmeric, salt, pepper, and rosemary.

4. Stir in mozzarella cheese and cook until the cheese is melted and thoroughly combined.

5. Serve topped with rosemary.

Nutrition:

- Calories 275

- Fat 17 g

- Carbohydrates 17.7 g

- Sugar 6.2 g

- Protein 12.6 g

- Cholesterol 45 mg

Vegan Cheesy Chips with Tomatoes

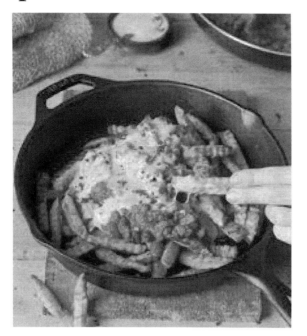

Preparation Time: 10 minutes

Cooking Time: 30 minutes

Servings: 6

Ingredients

- 5 tomatoes, sliced

- ¼ cup olive oil

- 1 tbsp chili seasoning mix

For vegan cheese

- ½ cup pepitas seeds

- 1 tbsp nutritional yeast

- Salt and black pepper, to taste

- 1 tsp garlic puree

Directions

1. Over the sliced tomatoes, drizzle olive oil. Set oven to 400°F.

2. In a food processor, add all vegan cheese ingredients and pulse until the desired consistency is attained.

3. Transfer to a bowl and stir in chili seasoning mix.

4. Toss in the tomato slices to coat.

5. Set the tomato slices on the prepared baking pan and bake for 10 minutes.

Mixed Veggie Salad

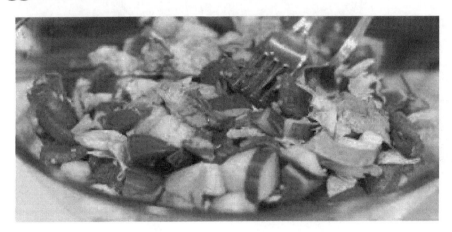

Preparation Time: 20 minutes

Cooking Time: 0 minutes

Servings: 6

Allergens: dairy

Ingredients:

For Dressing:

- 1 small avocado, peeled, pitted and chopped

- ¼ cup plain Greek yogurt

- 1 small yellow onion, chopped

- 1 garlic clove, chopped

- 2 tablespoons fresh parsley
- 2 tablespoons fresh lemon juice

For Salad:

- 6 cups fresh spinach, shredded
- 2 medium zucchinis, cut into thin slices
- ½ cup celery, sliced
- ½ cup red bell pepper, seeded and sliced thinly
- ½ cup yellow onion, sliced thinly
- ½ cup cucumber, sliced thinly
- ½ cup cherry tomatoes, halved
- ¼ cup Kalamata olives, pitted
- ½ cup feta cheese, crumbled

Directions:

1. For dressing: in a food processor, add all the ingredients and pulse until smooth.
2. For the salad: in a salad bowl, add all the ingredients and mix well.
3. Pour the dressing over salad and gently, toss to coat well.
4. Serve immediately.

Nutrition:

- Calories 592
- Fat 18.1 g
- Carbohydrates 88.4 g
- Sugar 5 g
- Protein 21.3 g
- Cholesterol 0 mg

Smoked Tofu with Rosemary Sauce

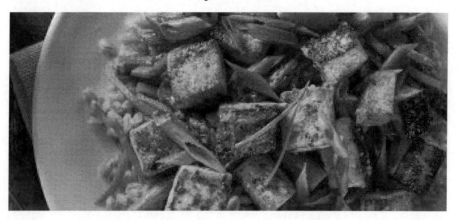

Preparation Time: 10 minutes

Cooking Time:20 minutes

Servings: 6

Ingredients

- 10 ounces smoked tofu

- 2 tbsp sesame oil

- 1 onion, chopped

- 1 tsp garlic, minced

- ½ cup vegetable broth

- ½ tsp turmeric powder

- Salt and black pepper, to taste

- For the sauce

- ½ tbsp olive oil

- 1 cup tomato sauce

- 2 tbsp white wine

- 1 tsp fresh rosemary, chopped

- 1 tsp chili garlic sauce

Directions

1. Pat dry the tofu using a paper towel and chop into 1-inch cubes. Set a frying pan over medium heat and warm sesame oil. Add in the tofu cubes and fry until browned.

2. Stir in salt, broth, black pepper, garlic, turmeric powder, and onions.

3. Cook until all liquid evaporates.

4. As the process goes on, you can prepare the sauce. Set a pan over medium heat and warm olive oil.

5. Place in tomato sauce and heat until cooked through.

6. Place in the rest of the ingredients and simmer for 10 minutes over medium heat.

7. Serve with prepared tofu cubes!

Nutrition:

- Calories: 290
- Carbohydrates: 10.6g
- Protein: 7.4g
- Fat: 25g
- Sugar: 4g
- Sodium: 1069mg

Deviled Eggs with Sriracha Mayo

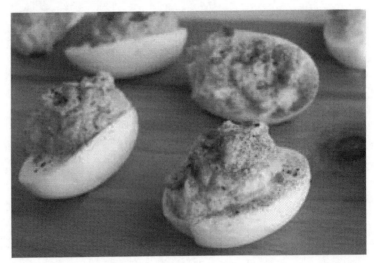

Preparation Time: 10 minutes

Cooking Time:30 minutes

Servings: 6

Ingredients

- 8 large eggs

- 3 cups water

- Ice water bath

- 3 tbsp sriracha sauce

- 4 tbsp mayonnaise

- Salt to taste

- ¼ tsp smoked paprika

Directions

1. Bring eggs to boil in salted water in a pot over high heat, and then reduce the heat to simmer for 10 minutes. Transfer eggs to an ice water bath, let cool completely and peel the shells.

2. Slice the eggs in half height wise and empty the yolks into a bowl. Smash with a fork and mix in sriracha sauce, mayonnaise, and half of the paprika until smooth.

3. Spoon filling into a piping bag with a round nozzle and fill the egg whites to be slightly above the brim.

4. Garnish with remaining paprika and serve.

Nutrition:

- Kcal 415
- Carbs 63g
- Fat 9g
- Protein 15g

Crunchy Pork Rind and Zucchini Sticks

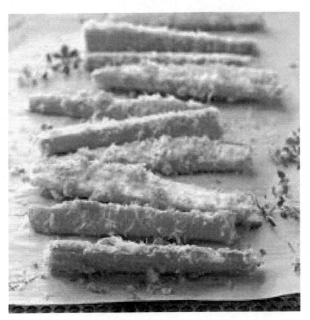

Preparation Time: 10 minutes

Cooking Time:30 minutes

Servings: 6

Ingredients

- ¼ cup pork rind crumbs

- 1 tsp sweet paprika

- ¼ cup shredded Parmesan cheese

- Salt and chili pepper to taste

- 3 fresh eggs

- 2 zucchinis, cut into strips

- Aioli:

- ½ cup mayonnaise

- 1 garlic clove, minced

- Juice and zest from ½ lemon

Directions

1. Preheat oven to 425°F and line a baking sheet with foil. Grease with cooking spray and set aside. Mix the pork rinds, paprika, Parmesan cheese, salt, and chili pepper in a bowl. Beat the eggs in another bowl.

2. Coat zucchini strips in eggs, then in Parmesan mixture, and arrange on the baking sheet. Grease lightly with cooking spray and bake for 15 minutes to be crispy.

3. To make the aioli, combine in a bowl mayonnaise, lemon juice, and garlic, and gently stir until everything is well incorporated. Add the lemon zest, adjust the seasoning, and stir again.

4. Cover and place in the refrigerator until ready to serve.

5. Serve the zucchini strips with garlic aioli for dipping.

Nutrition:

- Kcal 488
- Carbs 25g
- Fat 33g
- Protein 26g

Baked Cheese & Spinach Balls

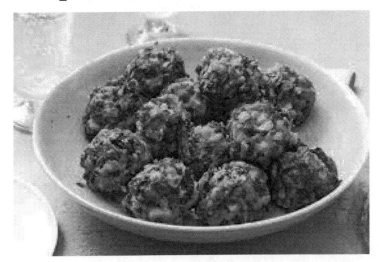

Preparation Time: 10 minutes

Cooking Time:10 minutes

Servings: 6

Ingredients

- ⅓ cup crumbled ricotta cheese

- ¼ tsp nutmeg

- ¼ tsp pepper

- 3 tbsp heavy cream

- 1 tsp garlic powder

- 1 tbsp onion powder

- 2 tbsp butter, melted

- ⅓ cup Parmesan cheese, shredded

- 2 eggs

- 1 cup spinach

- 1 cup almond flour

Directions

1. Place all ingredients in a food processor. Process until smooth. Place in the freezer for about 10 minutes.

2. Make balls out of the mixture and arrange them on a lined baking sheet.

3. Bake in the oven at 350°F for about 10-12 minutes.

Nutrition:

*   Kcal 345

*   Carbs 12g

*   Fat 18g

*   Protein 36g

Duo-Cheese Chicken Bake

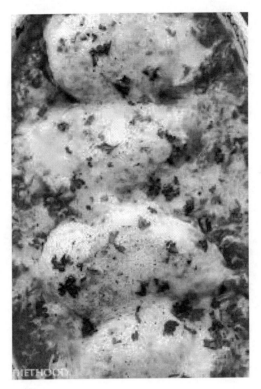

Preparation Time: 10 minutes

Cooking Time:40 minutes

Servings: 6

Ingredients

- 2 tbsp olive oil

- 8 oz cream cheese

- 1 lb. ground chicken

- 1 cup buffalo sauce

- 1 cup ranch dressing

- 3 cups grated yellow cheddar cheese

Directions

1. Preheat oven to 350°F. Lightly grease a baking sheet with a cooking spray. Warm the oil in a skillet over medium heat and brown the chicken for a couple of minutes, take off the heat, and set aside.

2. Spread cream cheese at the bottom of the baking sheet, top with chicken, pour buffalo sauce over, add ranch dressing, and sprinkle with cheddar cheese.

3. Bake for 23 minutes until cheese has melted and golden brown on top.

4. Remove and serve with veggie sticks or low carb crackers

Nutrition:

- Kcal 450

- Carbs 44g

- Fat 18g

- Protein 31g

Spicy Chicken Cucumber Bites

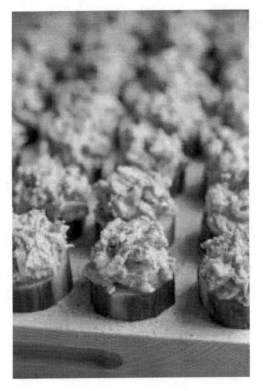

Preparation Time: 10 minutes

Cooking Time: 30 minutes

Servings: 6

Ingredients

- 2 cucumbers, sliced with a 3-inch thickness
- 2 cups small dices leftover chicken
- ¼ jalapeño pepper, seeded and minced
- 1 tbsp Dijon mustard
- ⅓ cup mayonnaise
- Salt and black pepper to taste

Directions

1. Cut mid-level holes in cucumber slices with a knife and set aside.

2. Combine chicken, jalapeno pepper, mustard, mayonnaise, salt, and black pepper to be evenly mixed.

3. Fill cucumber holes with chicken mixture and serve.

Nutrition:

- Kcal 429
- Carbs 49g
- Fat 22g
- Protein 11g

Cheesy Cauliflower Bake with Mayo Sauce

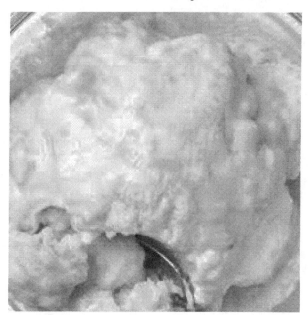

Preparation Time: 10 minutes

Cooking Time: 20 minutes

Servings: 6

Ingredients

- 2 heads cauliflower, cut into florets

- ¼ cup melted butter

- Salt and black pepper to taste

- 1 pinch red pepper flakes

- ½ cup mayonnaise

- ¼ tsp Dijon mustard

- 3 tbsp grated pecorino cheese

Directions

1. Preheat oven to 400°F and grease a baking dish with cooking spray.

2. Combine the cauli florets, butter, salt, black pepper, and red pepper flakes in a bowl until well mixed. Mix the mayonnaise and Dijon mustard in a bowl and set aside until ready to serve.

3. Arrange cauliflower florets on the prepared baking dish. Sprinkle with grated pecorino cheese and bake for 25 minutes until the cheese has melted and golden brown on the top.

4. Remove, let sit for 3 minutes to cool, and serve with the mayo sauce.

Nutrition:

- Calories 140

- Total Fats 1.5g

- Carbs: 15g

- Protein 7g

- Dietary Fiber: 3.2g

Zucchini Gratin with Feta Cheese

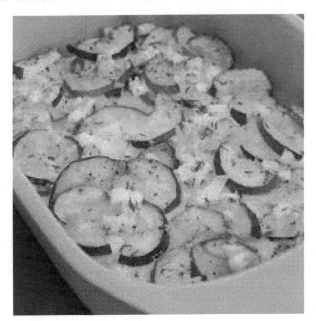

Preparation Time: 10 minutes

Cooking Time:20 minutes

Servings: 6

Ingredients

- 2 lb. zucchinis, sliced

- 2 red bell peppers, seeded and sliced

- Salt and black pepper to taste

- 1 ½ cups crumbled feta cheese

- 2 tbsp butter, melted

- ¼ tsp xanthan gum

- ½ cup heavy whipping cream

Directions

1. Preheat oven to 370ºF. Place the sliced zucchinis in a colander over the sink, sprinkle with salt and let sit for 20 minutes. Transfer to paper towels to drain the excess liquid.

2. Grease a baking dish with cooking spray and make a layer of zucchini and bell peppers overlapping one another. Season with pepper, and sprinkle with feta cheese. Repeat the layering process a second time.

3. Combine the butter, xanthan gum, and whipping cream in a bowl, stir to mix completely, and pour over the vegetables. Bake for 30-40 minutes or until golden brown on top.

Nutrition:

- Kcal 473

- Carbs 28g

- Fat 32g

- Protein 19g

Coconut Ginger Macaroons

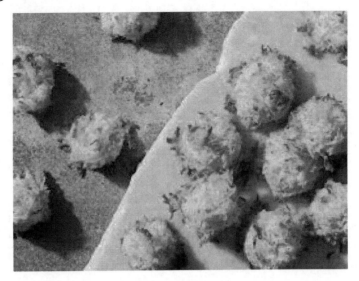

Preparation Time: 10 minutes

Cooking Time: 50 minutes

Servings: 6

Ingredients

- 2 fingers ginger root, pureed

- 6 egg whites

- 1 cup finely shredded coconut

- ¼ cup swerve

- A pinch of chili powder

- 1 cup water

- Angel hair chili to garnish

Directions

1. Preheat the oven to 350°F and line a baking sheet with parchment paper. Set aside.

2. In a heatproof bowl, whisk ginger, egg whites, coconut, swerve, and chili powder. Bring the water to boil in a pot over medium heat and place the heatproof bowl on the pot. Continue whisking the mixture until it is glossy, about 4 minutes.

3. Do not let the bowl touch the water or be too hot so that the eggs don't cook.

4. Spoon the mixture into the piping bag after and pipe out 40 to 50 little mounds on the lined baking sheet.

5. Bake the macaroons in the middle part of the oven for 15 minutes.

6. Once they are ready, transfer them to a wire rack, garnish them with the angel hair chili, and serve.

Nutrition:

- Kcal 330
- Carbs 11g
- Fat 28g
- Protein 14g

Cheesy Green Bean Crisps

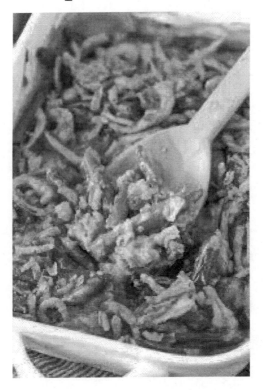

Preparation Time: 10 minutes

Cooking Time:40 minutes

Servings: 6

Ingredients

- ¼ cup pecorino Romano cheese, shredded
- ¼ cup pork rind crumbs
- 1 tsp garlic powder
- Salt and black pepper to taste
- 2 eggs
- 1 lb. green beans, thread removed

Directions

1. Preheat oven to 425°F and line two baking sheets with foil. Grease with cooking spray and set aside.

2. Mix the pecorino, pork rinds, garlic powder, salt, and black pepper in a bowl. Beat the eggs in another bowl.

3. Coat green beans in eggs, then cheese mixture and arrange evenly on the baking sheets.

4. Grease lightly with cooking spray and bake for 15 minutes to be crispy.

5. Transfer to a wire rack to cool before serving. Serve with sugar-free tomato dip.

Nutrition:

- Kcal 147
- Carbs 19g
- Fat 8g
- Protein 4g

Crispy Chorizo with Cheesy Topping

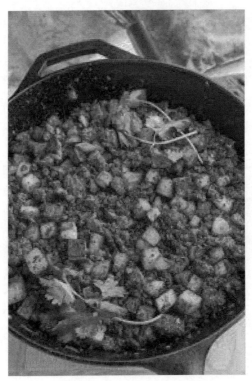

Preparation Time: 10 minutes

Cooking Time: 50 minutes

Servings: 6

Ingredients

- 7 ounces Spanish chorizo, sliced

- 4 ounces cream cheese

- ¼ cup chopped parsley

Directions

1. Preheat oven to 325°F. Line a baking dish with waxed paper. Bake chorizo for 15 minutes until crispy.

2. Remove and let cool. Arrange on a serving platter.

3. Top with cream cheese. Serve sprinkled with parsley.

Nutrition: Kcal 619 - Carbs 43g - Fat 35g - Protein 40g

Buttery Herb Roasted Radishes

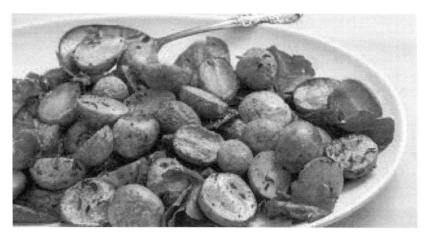

Preparation Time: 10 minutes

Cooking Time:40 minutes

Servings: 6

Ingredients

- 2 lb. small radishes, greens re moved
- 3 tbsp olive oil
- Salt and black pepper to season
- 3 tbsp unsalted butter
- 1 tbsp chopped parsley
- 1 tbsp chopped tarragon

Directions

1. Preheat oven to 400°F and line a baking sheet with parchment paper. Toss radishes with oil, salt, and black pepper. Spread on baking sheet and roast for 20 minutes until browned.

2. Heat butter in a large skillet over medium heat to brown and attain a nutty aroma, 2 to 3 minutes.

3. Take out the radishes from the oven and transfer to a serving plate. Pour over the browned butter atop and sprinkle with parsley and tarragon.

4. Serve with roasted rosemary chicken.

Nutrition: Kcal 435 - Carbs 20g - Fat 25g - Protein 38g

Bacon-Wrapped Jalapeño Peppers

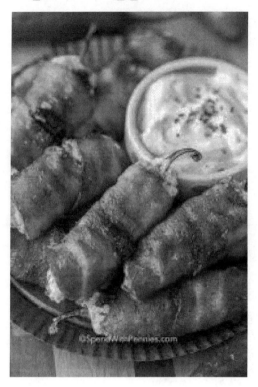

Preparation Time: 10 minutes

Cooking Time:40 minutes

Servings: 6

Ingredients

- 12 jalapeno peppers

- ¼ cup shredded Colby cheese

- 6 oz cream cheese, softened

- 6 slices bacon, halved

Directions

1. Cut the jalapeno peppers in half, and then remove the membrane and seeds. Combine cheeses and stuff into the pepper halves.

2. Wrap each pepper with a bacon strip and secure with toothpicks.

3. Place the filled peppers on a baking sheet lined with a piece of foil.

4. Bake at 350°F for 25 minutes until bacon has browned, and crispy and cheese is golden brown on the top.

5. Remove to a paper towel lined plate to absorb grease, arrange on a serving plate, and serve warm.

Nutrition:

- Calorie: 297
- Carbohydrates:6.2g
- Protein: 24.4g
- Fat: 20.1g
- Sugar: 2.7g
- Sodium: 479mg

Turkey Pastrami & Mascarpone Cheese Pinwheels

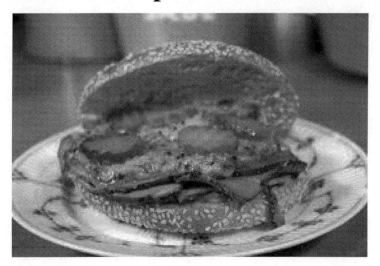

Preparation Time: 10 minutes

Cooking Time: 40 minutes

Servings: 6

Ingredients

- Cooking spray

- 8 oz mascarpone cheese

- 10 oz turkey pastrami, sliced

- 10 canned pepperoncini peppers, sliced and drained

Directions

1. Lay a 12 x 12 plastic wrap on a flat surface and arrange the pastrami all over slightly overlapping each other. Spread the cheese on top of the salami layers and arrange the pepperoncini on top.

2. Hold two opposite ends of the plastic wrap and roll the pastrami.

3. Twist both ends to tighten and refrigerate for 2 hours. Unwrap the salami roll and slice into 2-inch pinwheels. Serve.

Nutrition: Calorie: 140 - Carbohydrates: 15.3g - Protein: 6.5g - Fat: 6.2g - Sugar: 7.2g; Sodium: 1157mg

Garlicky Cheddar Biscuits

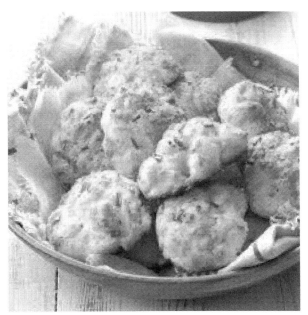

Preparation Time: 10 minutes

Cooking Time: 20 minutes

Servings: 6

Ingredients

- ⅓ cup almond flour
- 2 tsp garlic powder
- Salt to taste
- 1 tsp baking powder
- 5 eggs
- ⅓ cup butter, melted
- 1 ¼ cups grated sharp cheddar cheese
- ⅓ cup Greek yogurt

Directions

1. Preheat the oven to 350°F.

2. Mix the flour, garlic powder, salt, baking powder, and cheddar cheese, in a bowl.

3. In a separate bowl, whisk the eggs, butter, and Greek yogurt, and then pour the resulting mixture into the dry ingredients.

4. Stir well until a dough-like consistency has formed. Fetch half tbsp of the mixture onto a baking sheet with 2-inch intervals between each batter.

5. Bake for 12 minutes golden brown.

Nutrition:

- Calories 858
- Fat 48.1 g
- Carbohydrates 57.5 g
- Sugar 3 g
- Protein 47.3 g
- Cholesterol 164 mg

Roasted Stuffed Piquillo Peppers

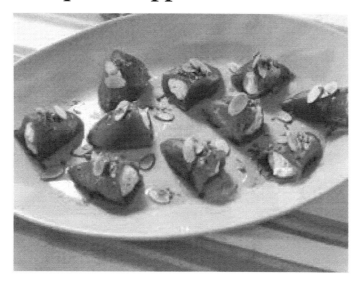

Preparation Time: 10 minutes

Cooking Time:30 minutes

Servings: 6

Ingredients

- 8 canned roasted piquillo peppers

- 1 tbsp olive oil

- 3 slices prosciutto, cut into thin slices

- 1 tbsp balsamic vinegar

Filling:

- 8 ounces goat cheese

- 3 tbsp heavy cream

- 3 tbsp chopped parsley

- ½ tsp minced garlic

- 1 tbsp olive oil

- 1 tbsp chopped mint

Directions

1. Mix all filling ingredients in a bowl. Place in a freezer bag, press down and squeeze, and cut off the bottom.

2. Drain and deseed the peppers. Squeeze about 2 tbsp of the filling into each pepper.

3. Wrap a prosciutto slice onto each pepper. Secure with toothpicks.

4. Arrange them on a serving platter. Sprinkle the olive oil and vinegar over.

Nutrition:

- Calories 525
- Total Fats 17g
- Carbs: 50g
- Protein 42g
- Dietary Fiber: 6g

Cream of Zucchini and Avocado

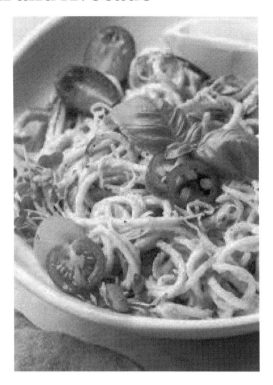

Preparation Time: 10 minutes

Cooking Time:20 minutes

Servings: 6

Ingredients

- 3 tsp vegetable oil

- 1 onion, chopped

- 1 carrot, sliced

- 1 turnip, sliced

- 3 cups zucchinis, chopped

- 1 avocado, peeled and diced

- ¼ tsp ground black pepper

- 4 cups vegetable broth

- 1 tomato, pureed

Directions

1. In a pot, warm the oil and sauté onion until translucent, about 3 minutes.

2. Add in turnip, zucchini, and carrot and cook for 7 minutes; add black pepper for seasoning.

3. Mix in pureed tomato, and broth; boil.

4. Change heat to low and allow the mixture to simmer for 20 minutes. Lift from the heat. Add the soup and avocado to a blender.

5. Blend until creamy and smooth.

Nutrition:

- Calories 640

- Total Fats 32g

- Carbs: 45g

- Protein 35g

- Dietary Fiber: 16g

Greek Salad with Poppy Seed Dressing

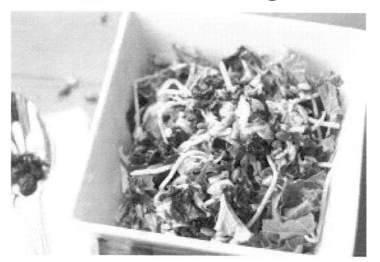

Preparation Time: 10 minutes

Cooking Time:30 minutes

Servings: 6

Ingredients

For the dressing

- 1 cup poppy seeds

- 2 cups water

- 2 tbsp green onions, chopped

- 1 garlic clove, minced

- 1 lime, freshly squeezed

- Salt and black pepper, to taste

- ¼ tsp dill, minced

- 2 tbsp almond milk

For the salad

- 1 head lettuce, separated into leaves

- 3 tomatoes, diced

- 3 cucumbers, sliced

- 2 tbsp kalamata olives, pitted

Directions

1. Put all dressing ingredients, except for the poppy seeds, in a food processor and pulse until well incorporated.

2. Add in poppy seeds and mix well with a fork.

3. Mix and divide salad ingredients between 4 plates. Add the dressing to each and shake to serve.

Nutrition:

- Calories 402

- Fat: 22.4g

- Carbohydrates: 16.3g

- Dietary Fiber: 6.83g

- Protein: 33.2g

Spicy Tofu with Worcestershire Sauce

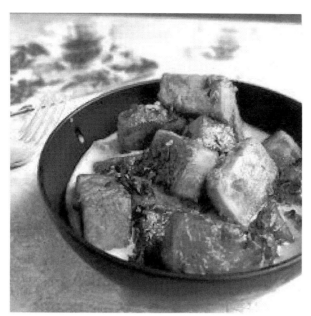

Preparation Time: 10 minutes

Cooking Time:20 minutes

Servings: 6

Ingredients

- 2 tbsp olive oil

- 14 ounces block tofu, pressed and cubed

- 1 celery stalk, chopped

- 1 bunch scallions, chopped

- 1 tsp cayenne pepper

- 1 tsp garlic powder

- 2 tbsp Worcestershire sauce

- Salt and black pepper, to taste

- 1 pound green cabbage, shredded

- ½ tsp turmeric powder

- ¼ tsp dried basil

Directions

1. Set a large skillet over medium heat and warm 1 tablespoon of olive oil. Stir in tofu cubes and cook for 8 minutes. Place in scallions and celery Cooking for 5 minutes until soft.

2. Stir in cayenne, Worcestershire sauce, pepper, salt, and garlic Cooking for 3 more minutes; set aside.

3. In the same pan, warm the remaining 1 tablespoon of oil. Add in shredded cabbage and the remaining seasonings and cook for 4 minutes. Mix in tofu mixture and serve warm.

Nutrition:

- Calories 237

- Fat: 8.53g

- Carbohydrates: 10.75g

- Dietary Fiber: 3.8g

- Protein: 8.54g

Cauliflower & Hazelnut Salad

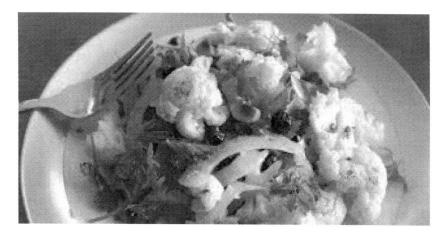

Preparation Time: 10 minutes

Cooking Time: 20 minutes

Servings: 6

Ingredients

- 1 head cauliflower, cut into florets

- 1 cup green onions, chopped

- 4 ounces bottled roasted peppers, chopped

- ¼ cup extra-virgin olive oil

- 1 tbsp wine vinegar

- 1 tsp yellow mustard

- Salt and black pepper, to taste

- ½ cup black olives, pitted and chopped

- ½ cup hazelnuts, chopped

Directions

1. Place the cauliflower florets in a steamer basket over boiling water. Cover and steam for 5 minutes; let cool and set aside. Add roasted peppers and green onions in a salad bowl.

2. Using a mixing dish, combine salt, olive oil, mustard, black pepper, and vinegar. Sprinkle the mixture over the veggies. Place in the reserved cauliflower and shake to mix well.

3. Top with hazelnuts and black olives and serve.

Nutrition:

- Calories 151

- Fat: 10.63g

- Carbohydrates: 13.75g

- Dietary Fiber: 1.2g

- Protein: 2.69g

Parsnip Chips with Avocado Dip

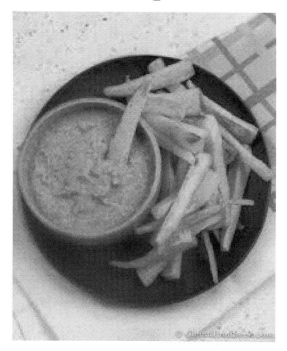

Preparation Time: 10 minutes

Cooking Time: 10 minutes

Servings: 6

Ingredients

- 2 avocados, pitted

- 2 tsp lime juice

- Salt and black pepper, to taste

- 2 garlic cloves, minced

- 2 tbsp olive oil

- For parsnip chips

- 3 cups parsnips, sliced

- 1 tbsp olive oil

- Salt and garlic powder, to taste

Directions

1. Use a fork to mash avocado pulp. Stir in fresh lime juice, pepper, 2 tbsp of olive oil, garlic, and salt until well combined.

2. Remove to a bowl and set the oven to 300°F.

3. Grease a baking sheet with spray.

4. Set parsnip slices on the baking sheet; toss with garlic powder, 1 tbsp of olive oil, and salt.

5. Bake for 15 minutes until slices become dry.

6. Serve alongside the well-chilled avocado dip.

Shrimp & Veggies Salad

An unforgettable and flavorsome salad of shrimp and fresh veggies...This delicious salad will be a great hit for summer entertaining.

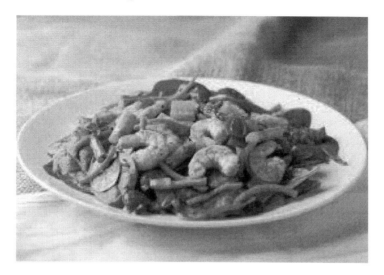

Preparation Time: 20 minutes

Cooking Time: 5 minutes

Servings: 6

Allergens: nuts

Ingredients:

For Dressing:

- 2 tablespoons natural almond butter

- 1 garlic clove, crushed

- 1 tablespoon fresh cilantro, chopped

- 2 tablespoons fresh lime juice

- 1 tablespoon yacon syrup

- ½ teaspoon cayenne pepper

- ¼ teaspoon salt

- 1 tablespoon water

- 1/3 cup olive oil

For Salad:

- 1 pound shrimp, peeled and deveined

- Salt and ground black pepper, as required

- 1 teaspoon olive oil

- 1 cup carrot, peeled and julienned

- 1 cup red cabbage, shredded

- 1 cup green cabbage, shredded

- 1 cup cucumber, julienned

- 4 cups fresh baby arugula

- ¼ cup fresh basil, chopped

- ¼ cup fresh cilantro, chopped

- 4 cups lettuce, torn

- ¼ cup almonds, chopped

Directions:

1. For dressing: in a bowl, add all ingredients except oil and beat until well combined.

2. Slowly, add oil, beating continuously until smooth.

3. For the salad: in a bowl, add shrimp, salt, black pepper, and oil and toss to coat well.

4. Heat a skillet over medium heat and cook shrimp for about 2 minutes per side.

5. Remove from the heat and set aside to cool.

6. In a large serving bowl, add all the cooked shrimp, remaining salad ingredients and dressing and toss to coat well.

7. Serve immediately.

Nutrition: Calories 273 - Fat: 22.32g - Carbs: 2.4g - Dietary Fiber: 1.1g - Protein: 15.3g

Caviar Salad

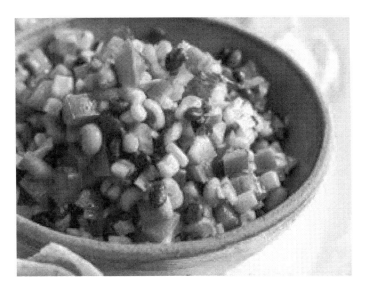

Preparation and Cooking time: 15 minutes

Servings: 12

Ingredients:

- 8 eggs, hard boiled, peeled and mashed with a fork

- 4 ounces black caviar

- 4 ounces red caviar

- Salt and black pepper to the taste

- 1 yellow onion, finely chopped

- ¾ cup mayonnaise

- Some toast baguette slices for serving

Directions:

1. In a bowl, mix mashed eggs with mayo, salt, pepper, and onion and stir well.

2. Spread eggs salad on toasted baguette slices, and top each with caviar.

Nutrition: Calories 231 - Fat 3.6 g - Carbohydrates 44.5 g - Sugar 1.7 g - Protein 5.8 g –

Cholesterol 0 mg

Caprese Salad

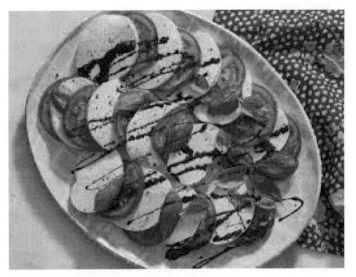

Preparation and Cooking Time: 7 minutes

Servings: 12

Ingredients:

- oz mozzarella cheese
- medium tomato
- basil leaves
- Salt and ground black pepper to taste
- teaspoon balsamic vinegar
- 1 tablespoon olive oil

Directions:

1. Slice mozzarella cheese and tomato. Torn basil leaves.
2. Alternate tomato and mozzarella slices on 2 plates.
3. Season with pepper and salt.
4. Drizzle vinegar and olive oil.
5. Sprinkle with the basil leaves.

Nutrition: Calories 110 - Total Fats - 10g Carbs - 6g Protein 3g - Dietary Fiber: 1g

Warm Asian Broccoli Salad

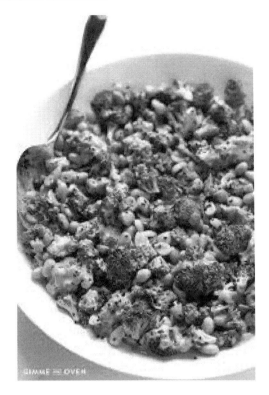

Preparation and Cooking Time: 15 minutes

Servings: 12

Ingredients:

- 12-ounce bag broccoli slaw
- ½ cup full fat plain goat milk yogurt
- 1 tsp fresh ginger, grated
- 2 tbsp coconut oil
- 1 tbsp coconut aminos
- ½ tbsp sesame seeds
- ½ tsp salt
- ¼ tsp pepper

- Cilantro as garnish, optional

Directions:

1. Add the coconut oil to a large skillet, and heat over medium-high flame.

2. Now add the broccoli slaw to the skillet.

3. Cover and cook for about 7 minutes.

4. Garnish with cilantro, if you desire.

5. Serve.

Nutrition:

- Calories – 346

- Fat – 18g

- Saturated Fat – 8g

- Trans Fat – 0g

- Carbohydrates – 26g

- Fiber – 3g

- Sodium – 576mg

- Protein – 27g

Warm Bacon Salad

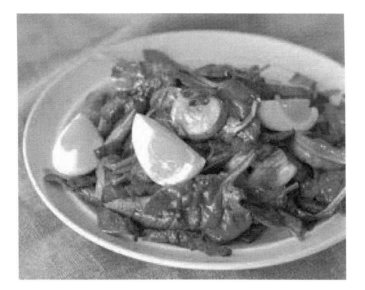

Preparation Time: 16 minutes

Cooking time: 18 minutes

Servings: 12

Ingredients:

- 16 oz bacon strips, chopped

- teaspoon cilantro

- 1 teaspoon ground ginger

- 1 teaspoon kosher salt

- tablespoon butter

- 4 boiled eggs, peeled and chopped

- 4 tomatoes, diced

- 1 oz spinach, chopped

- oz Cheddar cheese, grated

- 1 teaspoon almond milk

- oz eggplant, peeled and diced

Directions:

1. In medium bowl, combine bacon, cilantro, ginger, and salt.

2. Heat up pan over medium heat and melt 1 tablespoon of butter.

3. Put bacon in pan and cook for 5 minutes. Transfer bacon to plate.

4. Meanwhile, in bowl, mix together chopped eggs, tomatoes, and spinach.

5. Sprinkle with cheese and add almond milk.

6. Heat up pan again over medium heat and melt remaining 1 tablespoon of butter.

7. Add diced eggplants and fry for 8 minutes, stirring occasionally.

8. Then add bacon and roasted eggplants to salad.

9. Season with salt and stir gently.

10. Serve.

Nutritional Values

- Calories – 268

- Fat – 11g

- Saturated Fat – 4g

- Trans Fat – 0g

- Carbohydrates – 4g

- Fiber – 1g

- Sodium – 369mg

- Protein – 33g

Keto Avocado - Corn Salad

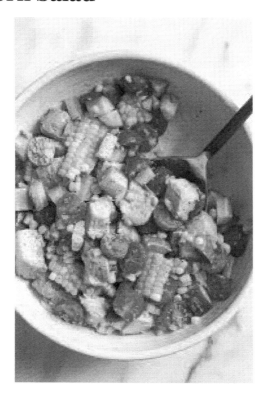

Preparation Time: 16 minutes

Cooking time: 18 minutes

Servings: 12

Ingredients Needed

The Salad:

- Cooked - corn on the cob - husk removed (1)
- Romaine head (1 chopped)
- Quartered grape tomatoes (4)
- Sliced red onion (.25 cup)
- Sliced avocado (half of 1)

The Dressing:

- Minced shallots (1 tbsp.)

- Dijon mustard (2 tsp.)

- White wine vinegar (2 tbsp.)

- 1% Vegan buttermilk (6 tbsp.)

- Garlic powder (.25 tsp.)

- Kosher salt (.5 tsp.)

- Black pepper (1 pinch)

- Extra-Virgin olive oil (2 tbsp.)

Directions:

1. Whisk each of the dressing components and place them in a serving jar.

2. Combine the salad fixings in a large salad bowl and toss with dressing.

Nutrition:

- Calories 428

- Fat: 42.65g

- Carbohydrates: 11.71

- Dietary Fiber: 3.4g

- Protein: 42.53g

Keto Cobb Salad

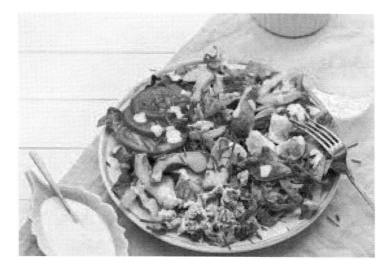

Preparation Time: 6 minutes

Cooking time: 30 minutes

Servings: 5

Ingredients Needed:

- Bacon strips (2)

- Hard-boiled egg (1)

- Spinach (1 cup)

- Campari tomato (half of 1)

- Chicken breast (2 oz.)

- Avocado (.25 of 1)

- Olive oil (1 tbsp.)

- White vinegar (.5 tsp.)

Directions

1. Fry the bacon and chicken. Shred or slice the chicken.

2. Cut all the fixings into small pieces.

3. Toss them to a bowl with the vinegar and oil. Toss gently and serve.

Nutrition: Calories 343 - Fat 9.1g - Carbs 46.8g - Sugar 3.4g - Protein 20g, Cholesterol 0mg

DESSERT

Eggless Strawberry Mousse

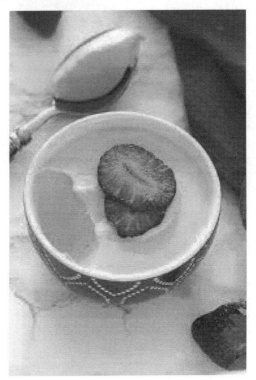

Preparation Time: 6 minutes

Cooking time: 30 minutes

Servings: 5

Ingredients

- 2 cups chilled heavy cream
- 2 cups fresh strawberries, hulled
- 5 tbsp erythritol
- 2 tbsp lemon juice
- ¼ tsp strawberry extract
- 2 tbsp sugar-free strawberry preserves

Directions

1. Beat the heavy cream, in a bowl, with a hand mixer at high speed until a stiff peak forms, for about 1 minute; refrigerate immediately.

2. Puree the strawberries in a blender and pour into a saucepan.

3. Add erythritol and lemon juice and cook on low heat for 3 minutes while stirring continuously.

4. Stir in the strawberry extract evenly, turn off the heat and allow cooling.

5. Fold in the whipped cream until evenly incorporated, and spoon into six ramekins.

6. Refrigerate for 4 hours to solidify.

7. Garnish with strawberry preserves and serve immediately.

Nutrition:

- Calories 347
- Fat 16.2 g
- Carbohydrates 43.8 g
- Sugar 10 g
- Protein 11.2 g
- Cholesterol 0 mg

Chocolate Chip Cookies

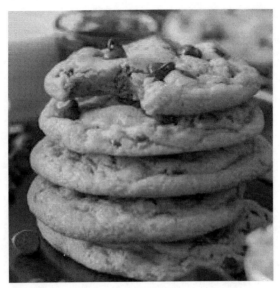

Preparation Time: 6 minutes

Cooking time: 40 minutes

Servings: 5

Ingredients

- 1 cup butter, softened

- 2 cups swerve brown sugar

- 3 eggs

- 2 cups almond flour

- 2 cups unsweetened chocolate chips

Directions

1. Preheat oven to 350°F and line a baking sheet with parchment paper.

2. Whisk the butter and sugar with a hand mixer for 3 minutes or until light and fluffy. Add the eggs one at a time and scrape the sides as you whisk.

3. Mix in almond flour at low speed until well combined.

4. Fold in the chocolate chips. Scoop 3 tablespoons each on the baking sheet creating spaces between each mound and bake for 15 minutes to swell and harden.

Nutrition:

- Calories 226

- Fat 14.3 g

- Carbohydrates 25.4 g

- Sugar 13.2 g

- Protein 4.3 g

- Cholesterol 0 mg

Coconut Bars

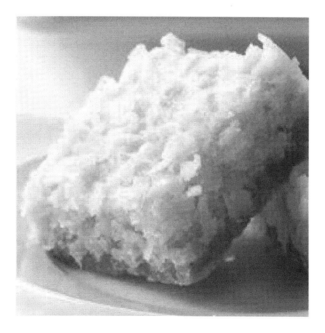

Preparation Time: 6 minutes

Cooking time: 40 minutes

Servings: 5

Ingredients

- 3 ½ ounces ghee

- 10 saffron threads

- 1 ⅓ cups coconut milk

- 1 ¾ cups shredded coconut

- 4 tbsp sweetener

- 1 tsp cardamom powder

Directions

1. Combine the shredded coconut with 1 cup of the coconut milk. In another bowl, mix together the remaining coconut milk with the sweetener and saffron. Let sit for 30 minutes.

2. Heat the ghee in a wok. Add the coconut mixtures and cook for 5 minutes on low heat, mixing continuously.

3. Stir in the cardamom and cook for another 5 minutes. Spread the mixture onto a small container and freeze for 2 hours.

4. Cut into bars and enjoy!

Nutrition:

- Calories 113

- Fat 3.1 g

- Carbohydrates 8.3 g

- Sugar 1.6 g

- Protein 12.3 g

- Cholesterol 31 mg

Berry Tart

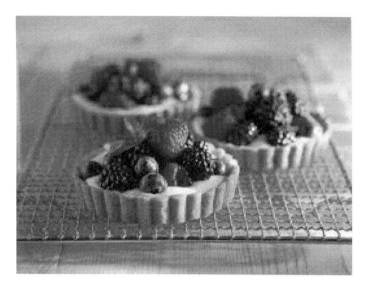

Preparation Time: 6 minutes

Cooking time: 30 minutes

Servings: 5

Ingredients

- 4 eggs

- 2 tsp coconut oil

- 2 cups berries

- 1 cup coconut milk

- 1 cup almond flour

- ¼ cup sweetener

- ½ tsp vanilla powder

- 1 tbsp powdered sweetener

- A pinch of salt

Directions

1. Preheat oven to 350°F. Place all ingredients except coconut oil, berries, and powdered sweetener, in a blender; blend until smooth. Gently fold in the berries.

2. Grease a baking dish with the oil. Pour the mixture into the prepared pan and bake for 35 minutes.

3. Sprinkle with powdered sugar to serve.

Nutrition:

- Calories 297

- Fat 20.5 g

- Carbohydrates 28.5 g

- Sugar 7.1 g

- Protein 3.9 g

- Cholesterol 0 mg

Creamy Hot Chocolate

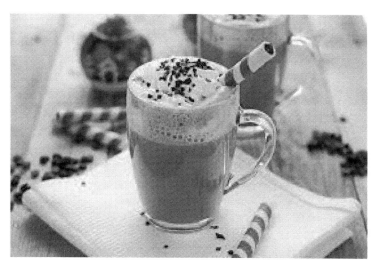

Preparation Time: 5 minutes
Cooking Time: 5 minutes
Servings: 4

Ingredients:

- 6 oz. dark chocolate, chopped
- ½ cup unsweetened almond milk
- ½ cup heavy cream
- 1 Tbsp. Erythritol
- ½ tsp vanilla extract

Directions:

1. Combine the almond milk, erythritol, and cream in a small saucepan. Heat it (choose medium heat and cook for 1-2 minutes).

2. Add vanilla extract and chocolate. Stir continuously until the chocolate melts.

3. Pour into cups and serve.

Nutrition: Kcal 314 - Carbs 19g - Fat 21g - Protein 13g

Delicious Coffee Ice Cream

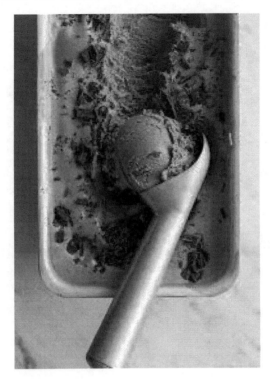

Preparation Time: 10 minutes
Cooking Time: 5 minutes
Servings: 1

Ingredients:

- 6 ounces coconut cream, frozen into ice cubes
- 1 ripe avocado, diced and frozen
- ½ cup coffee expresso
- 2 Tbsp. sweetener
- 1 tsp vanilla extract
- 1 Tbsp. water
- Coffee beans

Directions:

1. Take out the frozen coconut cubes and avocado from the fridge. Slightly melt them for 5-10 minutes.

2. Add the sweetener, coffee expresso, and vanilla extract to the coconut-avocado mix and whisk with an immersion blender until it becomes creamy (for about 1 minute).

3. Pour in the water and blend for 30 seconds.

4. Top with coffee beans and enjoy!

Nutrition:

- Kcal 858

- Carbs 51g

- Fat 52g

- Protein 47g

Easy Peanut Butter Cups

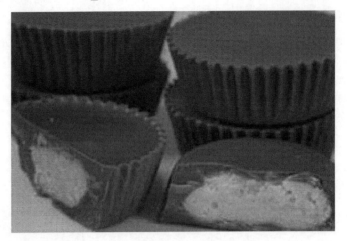

Preparation Time: 10 minutes
Cooking Time: 1 hour 35 minutes
Servings: 12 servings

Ingredients:

- 1/2 cup peanut butter

- 1/4 cup butter

- 3 oz. cacao butter, chopped

- 1/3 cup powdered swerve sweetener

- 1/2 tsp vanilla extract

- 4 oz. sugar-free dark chocolate

Direction:

1. Line a muffin tin with parchment paper or cupcake liners.

2. Using low heat, melt the peanut butter, butter, and cacao butter in a saucepan. Stir them until completely combined.

3. Add the vanilla and sweetener until there are no more lumps.

4. Carefully place the mixture in the muffin cups.

5. Refrigerate it until firm

6. Put the chocolate in a bowl and set the bowl in boiling water. This is done to avoid direct contact with the heat. Stir the chocolate until completely melted.

7. Take the muffin out of the fridge and drizzle in the chocolate on top. Put it back again in the fridge to firm it up. This should take 15 minutes to finish.

8. Store and serve when needed.

Nutrition:

- Calories 530

- Fat 21.2 g

- Carbohydrates 12.5 g

- Sugar 7.9 g

- Protein 69.6 g

- Cholesterol 201 mg

Raspberry Mousse

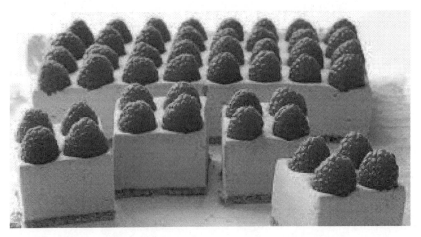

Preparation Time: 10 minutes
Cooking Time: 4 hours

Servings: 8

Ingredients:

- 3 oz. fresh raspberry

- 2 cups heavy whipping cream

- 2 oz. pecans, chopped

- ¼ tsp vanilla extract

- ½ lemon, the zest

Directions:

1. Pour the whipping cream into the dish and blend until it becomes soft.

2. Put the lemon zest and vanilla into the dish and mix thoroughly.

3. Put the raspberries and nuts into the cream mix and stir well.

4. Cover the dish with plastic wrap and put it in the fridge for 3 hours.

5. Top with raspberries and serve.

Nutrition: Calories 433 - Fat 20.8 g - Carbohydrates 12.3 g - Sugar 5.4 g - Protein 47.4 g Cholesterol 148 mg

Chocolate Spread with Hazelnuts

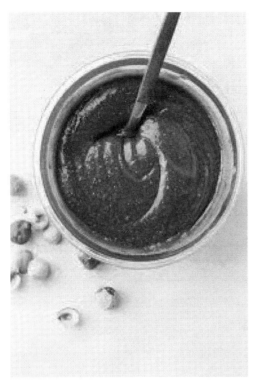

Preparation Time: 5 minutes
Cooking Time: 5 minutes
Servings: 6

Ingredients:

- 2 Tbsp. cacao powder

- 5 oz. hazelnuts, roasted and without shells

- 1 oz. unsalted butter

- ¼ cup of coconut oil

Directions:

1. Whisk all the spread ingredients with a blender for as long as you want.

2. Remember, the longer you blend, the smoother your spread.

Nutrition: Calories 440 - Total Fats 32g - Carbs: 12g - Protein 28g - Dietary Fiber: 2g

Quick and Simple Brownie

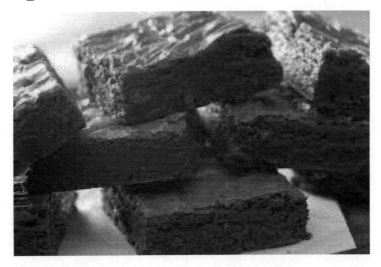

Preparation Time: 20 minutes
Cooking Time: 5 minutes
Servings: 2

Ingredients:

- 3 Tbsp. Keto chocolate chips

- 1 Tbsp. unsweetened cacao powder

- 2 Tbsp. salted butter

- 2¼ Tbsp. powdered sugar

Directions:

1. Combine 2 tbsp. of chocolate chips and butter, melt them in a microwave for 10-15 minutes. Add the remaining chocolate chips, stir, and make a sauce.

2. Add the cacao powder and powdered sugar to the sauce and whisk well until you have a dough.

3. Place the dough on a baking sheet, form the Brownie.

4. Put your Brownie into the oven (preheated to 350°F).

5. Bake for 5 minutes.

Nutrition: Calories 430 - Total Fats 38g - Carbs: 0g - Protein 22g - Dietary Fiber: 0g

Cute Peanut Balls

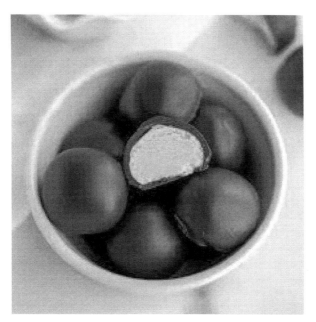

Preparation Time: 20 minutes
Cooking Time: 20 minutes
Servings: 18

Ingredients:

- 1 cup salted peanuts, chopped

- 1 cup peanut butter

- 1 cup powdered sweetener

- 8 oz keto chocolate chips

Directions:

1. Combine the chopped peanuts, peanut butter, and sweetener in a separate dish. Stir well and make a dough. Divide it into 18 pieces and form small balls. Put them in the fridge for 10-15 minutes.

2. Use a microwave to melt your chocolate chips.

3. Plunge each ball into the melted chocolate.

4. Return your balls in the fridge. Cool for about 20 minutes.

Nutrition: Calories 530 - Fat 19.3 g - Carbohydrates 10.5 g - Sugar 2.7 g - Protein 44.8 g Cholesterol 161 mg

Chocolate Mug Muffins

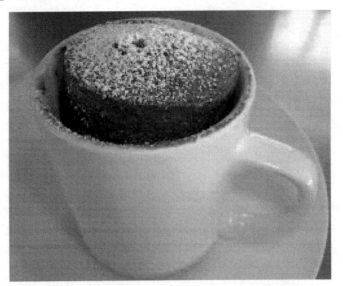

Preparation Time: 5 minutes
Cooking Time: 2 minutes
Servings: 4

Ingredients:

- 4 tbsps. almond flour

- 1 tsp baking powder

- 4 tbsp. granulated Erythritol

- 2 tbsp. cocoa powder

- ½ tsp vanilla extract

- 2 pinches salt

- 2 eggs beaten

- 3 tbsp. butter, melted

- 1 tsp coconut oil, for greasing the mug

- ½ oz. sugar-free dark chocolate, chopped

Directions:

1. Mix the dry ingredients in a separate bowl. Add the melted butter, beaten eggs, and chocolate to the bowl. Stir thoroughly.

2. Divide your dough into 4 pieces. Put these pieces in the greased mugs and put them in the microwave. Cook for 1-1.5 minutes (700 watts).

3. Let them cool for 1 minute and serve.

Nutrition:

- Calories 319
- Fat 13.5 g
- Carbohydrates 3.1 g
- Sugar 0.5 g
- Protein 44.1 g
- Cholesterol 136 mg

Blackcurrant Iced Tea

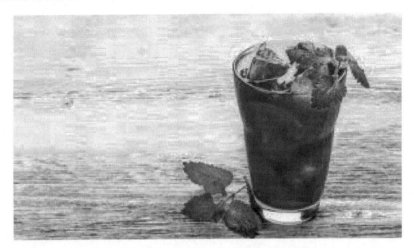

Preparation Time: 6 minutes

Cooking time: 30 minutes

Servings: 5

Ingredients

- 6 unflavored tea bags

- 2 cups water

- ½ cup sugar-free blackcurrant extract

- Swerve to taste

- Ice cubes for serving

- Lemon slices to garnish, cut on the side

Directions

1. Pour the ice cubes in a pitcher and place it in the fridge.

2. Bring the water to boil in a saucepan over medium heat for 3 minutes and turn the heat off. Stir in the sugar to dissolve and steep the tea bags in the water for 2 minutes.

3. Remove the bags after and let the tea cool down. Stir in the blackcurrant extract until well incorporated, remove the pitcher from the fridge, and pour the mixture over the ice cubes.

4. Let sit for 3 minutes to cool and after, pour the mixture into tall glasses.

5. Add some more ice cubes, place the lemon slices on the rim of the glasses, and serve the tea cold.

Nutrition:

- Calories 580

- Total Fats 40g

- Carbs: 2g

- Protein 49g

- Dietary Fiber: 1g

White Chocolate Cheesecake Bites

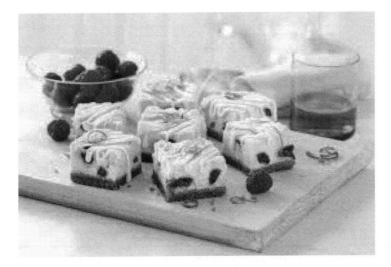

Preparation Time: 6 minutes

Cooking time: 30 minutes

Servings: 5

Ingredients

- 10 oz unsweetened white chocolate chips

- ½ half and half

- 20 oz cream cheese, softened

- ½ cup swerve

- 1 tsp vanilla extract

Directions

1. In a saucepan, melt the chocolate with half and a half on low heat for 1 minute. Turn the heat off.

2. In a bowl, whisk the cream cheese, swerve, and vanilla extract with a hand mixer until smooth. Stir into the chocolate mixture. Spoon into silicone muffin tins and freeze for 4 hours until firm.

Nutrition: Kcal 588 - Carbs 11g- Fat 35g - Protein 48g

Vanilla Chocolate Mousse

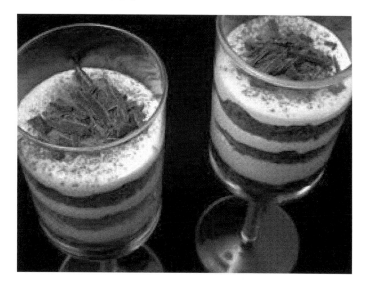

Preparation Time: 6 minutes

Cooking time: 30 minutes

Servings: 5

Ingredients

- 3 eggs

- 1 cup dark chocolate chips

- 1 cup heavy cream

- 1 cup fresh strawberries, sliced

- 1 vanilla extract

- 1 tbsp swerve

Directions

1. Melt the chocolate in a bowl, in your microwave for a minute on high, and let it cool for 10 minutes.

2. Meanwhile, in a medium-sized mixing bowl, whip the cream until very soft. Add the eggs, vanilla extract, and swerve; whisk to combine. Fold in the cooled chocolate.

3. Divide the mousse between four glasses, top with the strawberry slices and chill in the fridge for at least 30 minutes before serving.

Nutrition: Kcal 674 - Carbs 47g - Fat 31g - Protein 53g

Blueberry Ice Pops

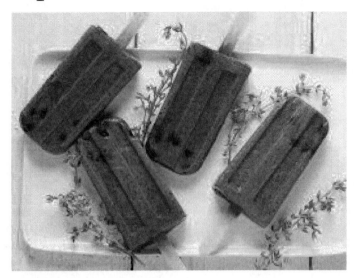

Preparation Time: 6 minutes

Cooking time: 30 minutes

Servings: 5

Ingredients

- 3 cups blueberries
- ½ tbsp lemon juice
- ¼ cup swerve
- ¼ cup water

Directions

1. Pour the blueberries, lemon juice, swerve, and water in a blender, and puree on high speed for 2 minutes until smooth.

2. Strain through a sieve into a bowl, discard the solids.

3. Mix in more water if too thick. Divide the mixture into ice pop molds, insert stick cover, and freeze for 4 hours to 1 week.

4. When ready to serve, dip in warm water and remove the pops.

Nutrition: Kcal 424 - Carbs 6g - Fat 31g; - Protein 31g

Strawberry Vanilla Shake

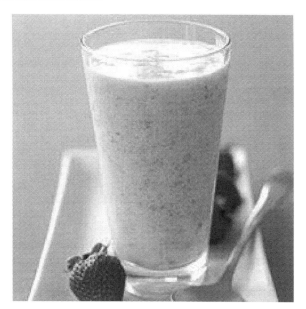

Preparation Time: 6 minutes

Cooking time: 30 minutes

Servings: 5

Ingredients

- 2 cups strawberries, stemmed an d halved
- 12 strawberries to garnish
- ½ cup cold unsweetened almond milk
- 2/3 tsp vanilla extract
- ½ cup heavy whipping cream
- 2 tbsp swerve

Directions

1. Process the strawberries, milk, vanilla extract, whipping cream, and swerve in a large blender for 2 minutes; work in two batches if needed.
2. The shake should be frosty.
3. Pour into glasses, stick in straws, garnish with strawberry halves, and serve.

Nutrition: Kcal 720 - Carbs 38g - Fat 42g - Protein 49g

Cranberry White Chocolate Barks

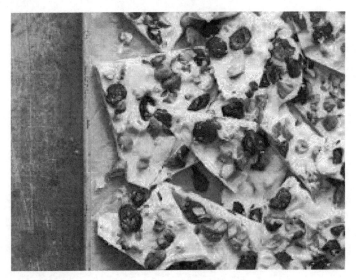

Preparation Time: 6 minutes

Cooking time: 30 minutes

Servings: 5

Ingredients

- 10 oz unsweetened white chocolate, chopped

- ½ cup erythritol

- ⅓ cup dried cranberries, chopped

- ⅓ cup toasted walnuts, chopped

- ¼ tsp pink salt

Directions

1. Line a baking sheet with parchment paper. Pour chocolate and erythritol in a bowl, and melt in the microwave for 25 seconds, stirring three times until fully melted.

2. Stir in the cranberries, walnuts, and salt, reserving a few cranberries and walnuts for garnishing.

3. Pour the mixture on the baking sheet and spread out. Sprinkle with remaining cranberries and walnuts. Refrigerate for 2 hours to set. Break into bite-size pieces to serve.

Nutrition: Kcal 537 - Carbs 15g - Fat 38g - Protein 33g

Vanilla Ice Cream

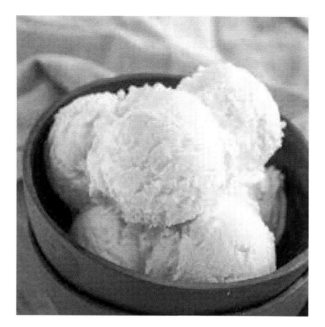

Preparation Time: 6 minutes

Cooking time: 30 minutes

Servings: 5

Ingredients

- ½ cup smooth peanut butter
- ½ cup swerve
- 3 cups half and half
- 1 tsp vanilla extract
- 2 pinches salt

Directions

1. Beat peanut butter and swerve in a bowl with a hand mixer until smooth. Gradually whisk in half and half until thoroughly combined.

2. Mix in vanilla and salt. Pour mixture into a loaf pan and freeze for 45 minutes until firmed up. Scoop into glasses when ready to eat and serve.

Nutrition: Calories 660 - Total Fats 50g - Carbs: 3g - Protein 47g - Dietary Fiber: 0.5g

Chia and Blackberry Pudding

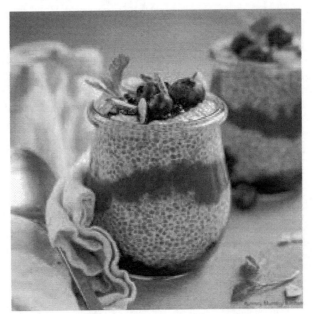

Preparation Time: 6 minutes

Cooking time: 30 minutes

Servings: 5

Ingredients

- 1 cup full-fat natural yogurt

- 2 tsp swerve

- 2 tbsp chia seeds

- 1 cup fresh blackberries

- 1 tbsp lemon zest

- Mint leaves, to serve

Directions

3. Mix together the yogurt and the swerve. Stir in the chia seeds. Reserve 4 blackberries for garnish and mash the remaining ones with a fork until pureed. Stir in the yogurt mixture

4. Chill in the fridge for 30 minutes.

5. When cooled, divide the mixture between 2 glasses.

6. Top each with a couple of blackberries, mint leaves, lemon zest and serve.

Nutrition:

- Kcal 490

- Carbs 21g

- Fat 27g

- Protein 41g

Mint Chocolate Protein Shake

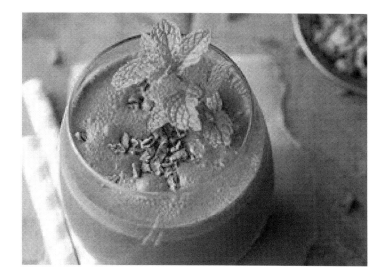

Preparation Time: 6 minutes

Cooking time: 50 minutes

Servings: 5

Ingredients

- 3 cups flax milk, chilled

- 3 tsp unsweetened cocoa powder

- 1 avocado, pitted, peeled, sliced

- 1 cup coconut milk, chilled

- 3 mint leaves + extra to garnish

- 3 tbsp erythritol

- 1 tbsp low carb Protein powder

- Whipping cream for topping

Directions

1. Combine the milk, cocoa powder, avocado, coconut milk, mint leaves, erythritol, and protein powder into a blender, and blend for 1 minute until smooth.

2. Pour into serving glasses, lightly add some whipping cream on top, and garnish with mint leaves.

Nutrition:

- Calories 324

- Fat 12.6 g

- Carbohydrates 9.7 g

- Sugar 5.5 g

- Protein 41.2 g

- Cholesterol 129 mg

Almond Butter Fat Bombs

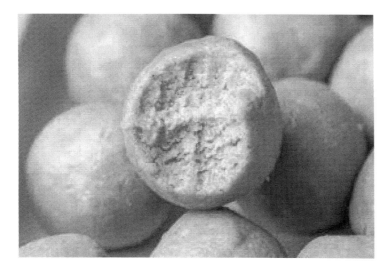

Preparation Time: 6 minutes

Cooking time: 30 minutes

Servings: 5

Ingredients

- ½ cup almond butter

- ½ cup coconut oil

- 4 tbsp unsweetened cocoa powder

- ½ cup erythritol

Directions

1. Melt butter and coconut oil in the microwave for 45 seconds, stirring twice until properly melted and mixed. Mix in cocoa powder and erythritol until completely combined.

2. Pour into muffin molds and refrigerate for 3 hours to harden.

Nutrition: Kcal 574- Carbs 10g - Fat 48g - Protein 28g

Almond Milk Hot Chocolate

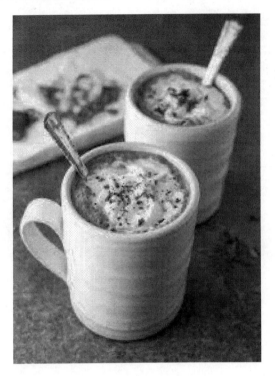

Preparation Time: 6 minutes

Cooking time: 30 minutes

Servings: 5

Ingredients

- 3 cups almond milk

- 4 tbsp unsweetened cocoa powder

- 2 tbsp swerve

- 3 tbsp almond butter

- Finely chopped almonds to garnish

Directions

1. In a saucepan, add the almond milk, cocoa powder, and swerve. Stir the mixture until the sugar dissolves.

2. Set the pan over low to heat through for 5 minutes, without boiling.

3. Swirl the mix occasionally.

4. Turn the heat off and stir in the almond butter to be incorporated. Pour the hot chocolate into mugs and sprinkle with chopped almonds.

5. Serve hot.

Nutrition:

- Calories 309

- Fat 18 g

- Carbohydrates 6.6 g

- Sugar 2.9 g

- Protein 29.7 g

- Cholesterol 77 mg

Berry Merry

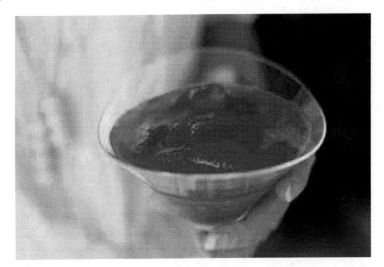

Preparation Time: 6 minutes

Cooking time: 30 minutes

Servings: 5

Ingredients

- 1 ½ cups blackberries

- 1 cup strawberries + extra for garnishing

- 1 cup blueberries

- 2 small beets, peeled and chopped

- 2/3 cup ice cubes

- 1 lime, juiced

Directions

1. For the extra strawberries for garnishing, make a single deep cut on their sides; set aside.

2. Add the blackberries, strawberries, blueberries, beet, and ice into the smoothie maker and blend the ingredients at high speed until smooth and frothy, for about 60 seconds.

3. Add the lime juice, and puree further for 30 seconds.

4. Pour the drink into tall smoothie glasses, fix the reserved strawberries on each glass rim, stick a straw in, and serve the drink immediately.

Nutrition:

- Kcal 284
- Carbs 12g
- Fat 12g
- Protein 31g

Coffee Fat Bombs

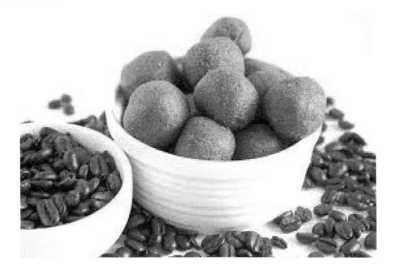

Preparation Time: 6 minutes

Cooking time: 30 minutes

Servings: 5

Ingredients

- 1 ½ cups mascarpone cheese
- ½ cup melted butter
- 3 tbsp unsweetened cocoa powder
- ¼ cup erythritol
- 6 tbsp brewed coffee, room temperature

Directions

1. Whisk the mascarpone cheese, butter, cocoa powder, erythritol, and coffee with a hand mixer until creamy and fluffy, for 1 minute.

2. Fill into muffin tins and freeze for 3 hours until firm.

Nutrition:

- Calories 413
- Fat 28.6 g
- Carbohydrates 7 g
- Sugar 1.8 g
- Protein 29.9 g
- Cholesterol 107 mg

Strawberry and Basil Lemonade

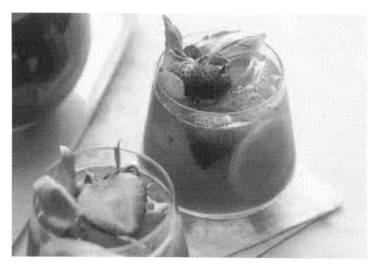

Preparation Time: 6 minutes

Cooking time: 30 minutes

Servings: 5

Ingredients

- 4 cups water

- 12 strawberries, leaves remove d

- 1 cup fresh lemon juice

- ⅓ cup fresh basil

- ¾ cup swerve

- Crushed Ice

- Halved strawberries to garnish

- Basil leaves to garnish

Directions

1. Spoon some ice into 4 serving glasses and set aside. In a pitcher, add the water, strawberries, lemon juice, basil, and swerve.

2. Insert the blender and process the ingredients for 30 seconds.

3. The mixture should be pink and the basil finely chopped. Adjust the taste and add the ice in the glasses.

4. Drop 2 strawberry halves and some basil in each glass and serve immediately.

Nutrition:

- Calories 620
- Fat 42.9 g
- Carbohydrates 10.5 g
- Sugar 2.7 g
- Protein 44.8 g

CHAPTER 5:

28-Day Meal Plan

DAYS	BREAKFAST	LUNCH	DINNER	DESSERT
1	Cheesy Sausage Quiche	Winter Cabbage and Celery Soup	Bacon Balls with Brie Cheese	Green Coconut Smoothie
2	Coconut Porridge	Spinach Soup with Shiitake mushrooms	Creamy Cheddar Deviled Eggs	Instant Coffee Smoothie
3	Bacon Omelet	Vegan Artichoke Soup	Jamon & Queso Balls	Keto Blood Sugar Adjuster Smoothie
4	Green Veggies Quiche	Seafood Soup	Cajun Crabmeat Frittata	Lime Spinach Smoothie
5	Chicken & Asparagus Frittata	Hot Spicy Chicken	Crabmeat & Cheese Stuffed Avocado	Protein Coconut Smoothie
6	Ricotta Cloud Pancakes with Whipped Cream	Broccoli and Turkey Dish	Juicy Beef Cheeseburgers	Strong Spinach and Hemp Smoothie
7	Mushroom & Cheese Lettuce Wraps	Easy Mayo Salmon	Cilantro & Chili Omelet	Green Low Carb Breakfast Smoothie

8	Bacon & Cheese Pesto Mug Cakes	Zesty Avocado and Lettuce Salad	Zucchini with Blue Cheese and Walnuts	Total Almond Smoothie
9	Mascarpone & Vanilla Breakfast Cups	Veggie, Bacon and Egg Dish	Garlick & Cheese Turkey Slices	Ultimate Green Mix Smoothie
10	Quickly Blue Cheese Omelet	Keto Teriyaki Chicken	Prosciutto & Cheese Egg Cups	The Strawberry Almond Smoothie
11	Breakfast Buttered Eggs	Low Carb Keto Pasta and Tomato sauce	Spanish Salsa Aioli	Early Morning Fruit Smoothie
12	Bacon & Cheese Zucchini Balls	Jamon & Queso Balls	Three-Cheese Fondue with Walnuts and Parsley	Banana Chai Smoothie with Cinnamon
13	Chorizo and Mozzarella Omelet	Lime Chicken with Coleslaw	Mushroom Salad	Berry Banana with Quinoa Smoothie
14	Hashed Zucchini & Bacon Breakfast	Spinach and Tuna Salad	Greek Side Salad	Eggless Strawberry Mousse
15	Morning Almond Shake	Rosemary Balsamic Chicken Liver Pate	Tomato Salsa	Chocolate Chip Cookies

16	Egg Omelet Roll with Cream Cheese & Salmon	Cheese and Bacon Stuffed Zucchini	Grilled Steak Salad	Coconut Bars
17	Traditional Spinach and Feta Frittata	Chicken and Greens Soup	Pork Burgers with Caramelized Onion Rings	Berry Tart
18	Chocolate Protein Coconut Shake	Cold Cauliflower and Cilantro Soup	Pork Chops with Cranberry Sauce	Creamy Hot Chocolate
19	Broccoli & Colby Cheese Frittata	Creamy Broccoli Soup with Nutmeg	Beef Pot Roast	Delicious Coffee Ice Cream
20	Baked Eggs in Avocados	Creamy Mushroom Soup with Crumbled Bacon	Beef Zucchini Cups	Easy Peanut Butter Cups
21	Ham and Vegetable Frittata	Creamy Mushroom and Zucchini Soup	Rosemary Balsamic Chicken Liver Pate	Raspberry Mousse
22	Eggs & Crabmeat with Creme Fraiche Salsa	Creamy Cauliflower Chowder	Skillet Chicken and Mushrooms	Chocolate Spread with Hazelnuts
23	Cheesy Sausage	Chicken Meatloaf Cups	Chicken with	Quick and

	Quiche	with Pancetta	Olive Tapenade	Simple Brownie
24	Coconut Porridge	Ham and Emmental Eggs	Creamy Chicken Casserole	Cute Peanut Balls
25	Bacon Omelet	Chorizo and Cheese Gofre	Garlic Chicken	Chocolate Mug Muffins
26	Green Veggies Quiche	Cheese, Ham and Egg Muffins	Pan–seared Duck Breast	Blackcurrant Iced Tea
27	Chicken & Asparagus Frittata	Baked Chicken Legs with Cheesy Spread	Sushi Shrimp Rolls	White Chocolate Cheesecake Bites
28	Ricotta Cloud Pancakes with Whipped Cream	Quatro Formaggio Pizza	Grilled Shrimp with Chimichurri Sauce	Vanilla Chocolate Mousse

CHAPTER 6:

Prohibited Products List

Sauces to Avoid

Barbecue sauce and various sugary condiments for salads ☐ Bread and baked goods: to reduce or eliminate the intake of whole meal bread, crackers, biscuits, white bread, sandwiches.

Pasta to Avoid

To be avoided because it is rich in carbohydrates ☐ Sweets: avoid ice cream, candy, and sweet baked goods ☐ Cereals: avoid wheat, rice, oats, and breakfast cereals ☐ Sweetened drinks: soda, fruit juice, sweetened tea, and sports drinks ☐ Vegetables: avoid those rich in starch such as potatoes, corn, peas, and pumpkin.

Legumes to Avoid

Avoid beans, chickpeas, lentils ☐ Alcoholic Beverages: Beer and sugary mixed drinks contain carbohydrates ☐ Fruits: avoid citrus fruits, grapes, bananas, and pineapples.

Grains to Avoid

Brown rice, white rice, oats, quinoa, amaranth, and bulgur.

Sweet Fruits to Avoid

Such as bananas, raspberry, dates, mangoes, tangerines, pear, and papaya,

Fish or pork that are factory farmed: Grain-fed meats, factory-farmed fish, salami, packed sausages, cured bacon, smoked meat, canned meat, corned beef, and cured meat

Artificial Sweeteners

White sugar, brown sugar, raw sugar, corn syrup, nectar, and other artificial sweeteners.

Refined Oils

Canola, margarine, peanut oil, sesame oil, safflower oil, and fast foods

Processed Snacks

Tortilla, whole wheat bread, and bagels, Ice cream, Baked foods such as cakes, candy, and muffins

Fat-free & Low-Fat Dairy

Fat-free cheeses, Sweetened yogurt, Low fat, and fat-free whole milk

Crackers & Chip

Potato chips, and all crackers

Sweet Drinks & Alcoholic

Wine, beer, flavored cocktails, and processed juice, tea, or coffee

Tropical, high carb fruits (like grapes, mango, and pineapple, etc.)

Juices (even 100% fruit juices)

Fats to Avoid

Avoid refined oils they contain omega-6 fatty acids which raise your blood pressure. Soybean oil, sunflower oil, peanut oil, corn oil, sesame oil, margarine, grape-seed oil. Also, avoid packed foods that contain processed Trans fats

Protein to Avoid

Avoid processed meats, packed sausage, canned meat, smoked meat, beef jerky, hotdogs, fatless cheese, sweetened yogurt, salami.

Carb to Avoid

Avoid starchy vegetables like potato, parsnip, beets, yucca, corn, peas, and sweet potato these vegetables are high in carb.

Avoid Fruits like mango, pear, dates, raisins, grapes, pineapple, apple are high in carb and sugar.

Avoid legumes and beans like black beans, kidney beans, fava beans, lima beans, chickpeas, pinto beans, oatmeal, lentils, and cereals. It contains high-carb values.

Avoid whole grains like wheat, rice, bulgur, quinoa, oat, barley, and buckwheat.

Sweeteners to Avoid

Avoid maple syrup, agave nectar, honey, sugar, corn syrup, sucralose, and Splenda.

CONCLUSION

Congratulations for making it this far! By now, I trust you already have a good understanding of the Ketogenic Diet and how it applies to you as you enjoy your 50s. Obviously, our goal here is to provide a Keto Diet guideline that works for you, taking into account your unique situation so that the best and most effective results can be achieved.

The ketogenic diet is one that has many important aspects and information that you need to know as someone who wants to try this diet. It is important to remember the warning that we have given you at the beginning of the book that this is not a diet that is safe and that doctors don't recommend to try it, and if you are going to attempt it remember that you shouldn't do so for longer than six months and even then never without the constant supervision of a doctor or at the very least a doctor knowing that you're doing this and that you're following their guidelines and words to the letter so they can make sure you are safe.

The ketogenic diet is a diet that believes that by minimizing your carbs while maximizing the good fat in your system while making sure that you're getting the protein you need; you will be happier and healthier. In this guidebook, we give you the information to know what this diet is all about, as well as describing the different types and areas that this diet will offer. Most people assume that there is only one way to do this and while there is one thing that the additional options share, there are four different options you can choose from. Each one has its unique benefits, and you should know about each type to learn what would be best for your body, which is why we have described them in the book for you to have the best information possible when you begin this diet for yourself.

Another important thing about this diet is that many people don't understand the importance of exercise with this diet. The best way to become healthier is to do three things for yourself. Get the right amount of sleep, eat healthily, and make sure that you get the proper amount of exercise as well for your body to work at an optimum level. The exercises, such as the ones that we explained, are the best to go with your diet to make sure that you are getting the most out of it.

For women who are on the go and have a busy lifestyle, we have provided recipes for a thirty-day meal plan so that you can make food quickly and have a great meal for their lifestyles. They also have enough servings for you to have leftovers so that you don't have to worry about preparing more food in the morning. Instead, you can simply pack it up and take it with you wherever you go. This works out so much easier for so many people because they don't have to cook in the morning, and it saves a busy person a lot of time.

With all this information at your fingertips, you will be able to enjoy this diet and use it to your advantage. Another benefit that we offer is that we explain routines that you can do for yourself to make this diet last longer for you and to benefit your body better as a result. Routines are very important and can be a big help to your body but also your spirit and your mind. Good luck with your keto journey!

One of the easiest ways to stay on your plan is to minimize the temptations. Remove the chocolate, candy, bread, pasta, rice, and sugary sodas you have supplied in your kitchen. If you live alone, this is an easy task. It is a bit more challenging if you have a family. The diet will also be useful for them if you plan your meals using the recipes included in this book.

If you cheat, that must count also. It will be a reminder of your indulgence, but it will help keep you in line. Others may believe you are obsessed with the plan, but it is your health and wellbeing that you are improving.

When you go shopping for your ketogenic essentials be sure you take your new skills, a grocery list, and search the labels. Almost every food item in today's grocery store has a nutrition label. Be sure you read each of the ingredients to discover any hiding carbs to keep your ketosis in line. You will be glad you took the extra time.

One significant motivation behind why we get so disappointed with standard weight control plans is that they regularly become misjudged and accomplish more damage than anything else.

So, in case you're needing a little motivation to read the book again, simply don't be excessively hard on yourself on the off chance that you miss a class or enjoy somewhat more than you needed. With these statements, you will realize that disappointment is part to remember the procedure.

But I think the most important thing I want you to learn from this book is this: it's never too late to make that change! It's never too late to try something new for self-improvement!

Made in the USA
Columbia, SC
11 January 2021